S0-ABY-265

THE MENTALLY
DISORDERED OFFENDER

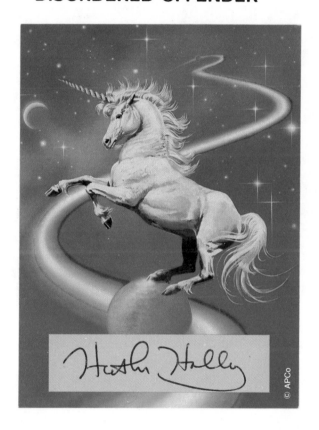

National Institute of Mental Health

THE MENTALLY
DISORDERED OFFENDER

Seymour L. Halleck, M.D.

Department of Psychiatry
University of North Carolina Memorial Hospital
Chapel Hill, North Carolina

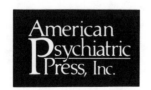

1400 K Street, N.W.
Washington, DC 20005

Books published by the American Psychiatric Press, Inc., represent the views and opinions of the individual authors and do not necessarily reflect the policies and opinions of the Press or the American Psychiatric Association.

This document was prepared under contract #81M052472101D awarded by the National Institute of Mental Health. Saleem A. Shah, Ph.D., served as the NIMH project officer.

The views expressed in this monograph are those of the author and do not necessarily reflect the official position of the National Institute of Mental Health or any other part of the U.S. Department of Health and Human Services.

The U.S. Government does not endorse or favor any specific commercial product. Trade or proprietary names appearing in this publication are used only because use was considered necessary by the author.

All material appearing in this volume except quoted passages from copyrighted sources is in the public domain and may be reproduced or copied without permission from the Institute or author. Citation of the source is appreciated.

First American Psychiatric Press edition published 1987

Manufactured in the United States

CONTENTS

FOREWORD

THIS MONOGRAPH FOCUSES ATTENTION on a number of legal and clinical issues at the interface of the criminal justice and mental health systems. Mentally ill persons who come into contact with the criminal process pose many challenges and problems to both systems since, at almost every stage, the nature of mental health evaluations and the delivery of care and treatment tend to be constrained and influenced by the particular legal rules and administrative requirements of the criminal justice agencies. Also, there is an all-too-common assumption that criminal defendants who are mentally ill—regardless of the nature of the alleged offense—are more likely to be dangerous and thereby warrant detention. Thus, even though defendants with a variety of serious criminal charges are typically free on bail pending trial, those considered to be mentally ill are very likely to be confined to secure mental health facilities while undergoing mental evaluations. The legal principle of using the "least restrictive alternative" for such evaluations is much more often found in statutory provisions and scholarly writings than in actual practice.

In this monograph Dr. Seymour A. Halleck, one of the leading psychiatrists in the country, provides an informative and provocative overview of the various categories of mentally ill offenders and of the salient legal and clinical issues that arise at the several stages of the criminal process. The monograph is designed for a wide and general audience and provides a very useful description and explication of a variety of difficult and longstanding problems. To this task Dr. Halleck brings more than 30 years of relevant experience. Clearly, his interest and knowledge in this area are substantially more than simply academic. Moreover, his writing reflects a deep and abiding concern for a class of individuals whose mental health and related needs are often overlooked and typically underserved in our society.

Saleem A. Shah, Ph.D.
Chief, Antisocial and Violent Behavior Branch
National Institute of Mental Health

PREFACE

THE STUDY OF BOTH CRIME and mental aberration deals with the interaction of many biological, psychological, and sociological variables. When criminal behavior and mental aberration coexist, as they usually do in the mentally disordered offender, the issues raised are so numerous that a monograph on the subject could discuss almost any aspect of criminal law or the behavioral sciences. I have selected for review only what, in my judgment, are the most critical issues.

This monograph begins by defining mentally disordered offenders and the problem of differentiating them from other offenders in terms of both treatment and housing. Next, a brief chapter describes society's three main objectives in dealing with offenders. These objectives receive different degrees of emphasis over time, and increased emphasis on any objective may be associated with diminished concern with the others. Consideration of the prevailing objectives helps the student of this subject understand societal responses to all classes of mentally disordered offenders.

Chapters 3 through 6 deal with the main classes of mentally disordered offenders. Each chapter begins with a description of how a particular class of mentally disordered offender is identified by the criminal justice system and a critical examination of some of the legal theories that justify its diversion from that system. The next section reviews some of the theoretical and practical issues of special concern to clinicians who must diagnose, treat, or care for that particular class of mentally disordered offender. Each chapter concludes with a brief review of emerging legal issues.

The description of the process by which mentally disordered offenders are identified sets the stage for considering more controversial issues. Some of the more difficult legal issues discussed are:

● The extent to which current notions of competency to stand trial accurately and fairly identify and divert those who are severely handicapped as they proceed through the criminal justice process.

- Whether the basic needs of the criminal justice system are served by identifying those who are not to be held criminally responsible for their crimes.
- Whether the legal concept of insanity can be conceptualized in practical or operational terms.
- Whether the concept of dangerousness should be used to justify differential treatment of offenders.
- How the criminal justice system defines the concept of mental disorder and the influence this definition has on its approach to the majority of offenders.

Some of the clinical issues discussed include:

- The skill of mental health specialists in assessing such qualities as pretrial competence, criminal responsibility, or dangerousness.
- The proper role of mental health specialists in making and communicating their assessments to the criminal justice system.
- The practices of the criminal justice system that complicate and sometimes impair the clinician's capacity to evaluate or treat mentally disordered offenders.

Some of the emerging legal issues considered include:

- The proper disposition for those who have been found incompetent to stand trial and whose competency appears unrestorable.
- The most useful and humane disposition for the insanity acquittee.
- The future of indeterminate sentencing programs.
- How the rights of offenders who have become mentally disturbed in prison can best be protected.

Chapter 7 deals with the treatment of mentally disordered offenders. A review of currently available treatment is presented and some of its deficiencies are considered.

Chapter 8 is a brief review of the ethical problems faced by clinicians who work with mentally disordered offenders. There is also a general discussion of how those ethical considerations may influence the present and future use of rehabilitative efforts, including the newly developed biological techniques for altering human behavior.

The final chapter is devoted to the issue of reform of the criminal justice system's handling of mentally disordered offenders. Two major questions are considered. First, what reforms would be desirable if the current philosophy of the criminal justice system remained unchanged? Second, would major changes in the basic philosophy of the criminal justice system better serve society's objectives in dealing with the crime problem in general and mentally disordered offenders in particular? I believe that the answer to the second question should be a qualified "yes." There are good reasons for modifying our current philosophy of corrections in the direction of emphasizing rehabilitation more and retribution less. To the extent that such a system is accepted, the problem of mentally disordered offenders becomes less special, and the principles that govern many aspects of their disposition become relevant to the criminal justice system as a whole.

CHAPTER 1

Which Offenders Are
Mentally Disordered?

MENTALLY DISORDERED OFFENDERS are formally identified on the basis of two general criteria. First, the evidence that they have committed a crime must be sufficient to lead to their arrest and arraignment. Second, an agency of the criminal justice system must suspect that they have a mental disorder of such proportion as to question the fairness or utility of subjecting them to the usual criminal justice process.

The first criterion expands the class of mentally disordered offenders to include some who have not been convicted of a crime. Defendants found incompetent to stand trial and those found not guilty by reason of insanity are not proven offenders. They are included here because they are believed to be emotionally disturbed and the evidence of their illegal activity is sufficient to convince key functionaries in the criminal justice system that they should be controlled by criminal or civil courts.

The second criterion requires that the mental disorder of offenders be apparent to those who manage the criminal justice system. Offenders who can conceal their distress or disability from authorities may never be labeled as disordered. Even if their incapacities are noted, that appellation is given only when officials in the judicial or correctional process conclude that their mental disabilities are of sufficient severity to justify their being treated in a substantially different manner from other offenders. Differential treatment by or even diversion from the criminal justice process is formalized when mentally disordered offenders are judged incompetent to proceed in the criminal process, not guilty by reason of insanity, "guilty but mentally ill," dangerous and in need of specialized treatment, or incapable of surviving in prison without a period of hospitalization.

Mentally disordered offenders constitute 5 to 6 percent of the total population of those institutionalized by virtue of some interaction with the criminal justice system (Monahan and Steadman 1983). Though relatively few, their importance to our system of correctional justice is disproportionately large. Their special designation and treatment by the criminal justice system raises fundamental questions about the nature of crime and punishment. Mentally disordered offenders also focus society's attention on the extent to which individual differences among offenders should be considered in the process of punishment, restraint, or treatment.

The criminal justice system does not regularly concern itself with psychological variables when dealing with ordinary offenders. Most offenders are assumed to be rational beings with sufficient capacity to respond to social sanctions or to survive the ordeal of trial and punishment. Before close attention is paid to disorders of mental functioning, a threshold level of mental impairment must be exceeded. As a rule, society does not judge that threshold to have been crossed unless the disability of offenders is severe.

By considering the influence of psychological variables on dispositional issues only when offenders are severely disabled, the criminal justice system spares itself a great deal of decision making. Once offenders are assumed to fall below a threshold of psychological impairment that calls for specialized treatment, their disposition can be determined without considering their psychological characteristics. Their impairments, however severe, are no longer relevant to criminal justice system decisions. By providing specific criteria for identifying and diverting abnormal offenders from its usual dispositions, the criminal justice system also affirms the "normality" of the majority of offenders who are not identified or diverted. Stone's (1975) description of the insanity defense as "the exception that proves the rule" can be generalized to include all the processes that divert mentally disordered offenders from the usual criminal justice dispositions. Once a form of incapacity is identified as an aspect of a mental disorder that justifies diversion, the criminal justice system can deal with all other offenders who are not diverted as though they were free of that type of impairment.

If mentally disordered offenders are to be viewed as "exceptions that prove the rule," their number must be carefully monitored. The size of the group must be kept large enough to ensure that they receive specialized care. At the same time, the size must be kept small enough to preserve the assumption that those who are diverted are truly "special" and that the others are without significant impairment.

Throughout this monograph I will question the fairness or efficiency of a system of criminal justice that draws a sharp line between mentally disordered and all other offenders. Here, I wish to simply assert that it is extremely difficult to draw such a line on a scientific or clinical basis. Offenders as a group differ in their capacity to meet criteria that define competency, sanity, mental illness, or dangerousness. The psychological variations that determine these capacities are distributed throughout the criminal population on a continuum that approximates a bell-shaped curve. This means that many who are not designated as mentally disordered offenders may have impairments just a little less severe than those who are. The size of the group that falls just below the threshold of impairment, which would justify special treatment, may in fact be quite large.

Mentally Disordered Offenders Who Are Not Formally Categorized

While this monograph deals primarily with formally designated mentally disordered offenders, those who work in correctional and security hospital settings must deal with many emotionally disturbed offenders who are never formally categorized as such. This group of individuals may share many characteristics with formally designated mentally disordered offenders. Both groups, for example, may experience similar degrees of distress and disability. But the two groups are managed quite differently by the criminal justice system. Those not formally designated as mentally disordered may go unnoticed by correctional authorities; if they are treated the usual purpose is to alleviate their suffering or help them adjust to a particular environment. No specific legal purpose underlies their treatment, such as restoring their competency or rehabilitating them, and those who treat them do not usually report their progress to judicial agencies.

Noncategorized Mentally Disordered Offenders in Prison

Determining which imprisoned offenders are suffering from mental disorders and need treatment is difficult. Our criminal justice system has a tradition of not designating certain diagnostic categories, viz., those disorders recognized by the official Diagnostic and Statistical Manual (DSM-III) of the American Psychiatric Association (1980), as true mental disorders. Thus, offenders with severe alcohol abuse problems or personality disorders are unlikely to be viewed as mentally disordered offenders unless they have other problems as well. The reasons for ignoring official psychiatric nomenclature are considered in a subsequent chapter. It is important to note, however, that if ordinary standards of diagnoses were used in the criminal justice system, the majority of offenders would probably be classified as mentally disordered.

An estimated 15 to 20 percent of incarcerated offenders need psychiatric treatment at some time during their imprisonment (Roth 1980). While this approximates the treatment needs of the general population, individuals who sorely need treatment but who wish to avoid being designated as mentally disordered probably find it easier to disguise their symptoms in prison. The routine of prison life and in particular the degree of isolation it imposes upon inmates allows seriously disordered offenders, including many who may be psychotic, to go undetected. On several occasions I have been asked to examine allegedly normal inmates for research or legal purposes and discovered that these individuals were floridly psychotic. These were offenders whose blatant hallucinations and delusions simply had not been noticed by prison authorities. My experience is not unique. Roth (1980) noted that correctional psychiatrists often encounter severely disturbed but untreated inmates within prisons and jails. If blatant psychosis can be hidden or undetected in prison, severe depression, which is much easier to conceal, is probably even more prevalent.

Even when correctional officials are aware of the mental disturbances of prisoners, they have several ways to deal with these persons without labeling them as mentally disordered. Many prisons have their own hospital units that provide treatment for disturbed offenders, even those who may be psychotic. When offenders are treated in the institution in which they were originally confined they are not, as a rule, formally designated as mentally disordered.

Imprisoned offenders with less serious mental disorders may come to the attention of the authorities and receive some type of brief treatment, usually classified under the rubric of counseling or crisis intervention. The offenders who make up this group may not be seriously incapacitated, but they experience episodes of anxiety or depression of sufficient severity to be classified as mentally disordered outside the criminal justice setting.

In most large prisons, certain administrative settings are characterized by a high prevalence of unlabeled mental disorder. One of these is the punitive segregation unit. Since prison authorities do not readily define rule-breaking behavior as a symptom of a mental disorder, even offenders who have so many adjustment problems that they serve most of their sentences in a segregated unit may not be viewed as mentally disturbed. If they behave irrationally while segregated, their conduct may be viewed as a regrettable but understandable response to their restricted environment. At the same time, more progressive institutions pay a good deal of attention to the psychological needs of these inmates. They may be given both group and individual counseling on the assumption that their deviant behavior is a sign of a mental disorder as well as a response to a stressful environment (Toch 1981). If psychiatrists are available to examine individuals who frequently occupy punitive segregation units, they usually discover a high incidence of psychosis and major affective disorder.

Protective custody is another setting in which mental disorder is likely to be prevalent. In the last three decades, most correctional facilities have created units that offer protection for inmates who claim that they cannot survive in the regular prison population. Usually inmates request protective custody because they fear rape or other types of assault. Conditions in these units tend to be almost as restrictive as those in punitive segregation. A harsh environment is believed necessary to discourage inmates from "dropping out" of the regular institutional population. Protective custody inmates may also be targeted for special counseling and treatment to help them deal with their restricted environment and to help them overcome personal vulnerabilities that make them fear assault. From my own experiences in evaluating and working with persons in such units, the personal vulnerabilities of many of these inmates are best described as manifestations of serious mental disorders.

Recent trends in mental health law may have led to an increase in the number of mentally disturbed individuals who end up in prison. As the criteria for civil commitment have become more stringent, more mentally ill people with only marginal ability to care for themselves have been left free to roam the streets. Often these individuals commit minor crimes and become clients of the criminal justice system (Slovenko and Luby 1974). Most professionals who work in the correctional system, especially in jails, believe they are now seeing a greater number of offenders who would in past years have been labeled mentally disordered and sent to hospitals. The number of these individuals eventually designated as mentally disordered offenders is unknown, but probably many are not.

Noncategorized Mentally Disordered Offenders in Hospital Settings

Severely disturbed offenders who are never formally categorized as mentally disordered can be found in settings other than prisons or security hospitals. Some individuals who commit minor offenses are informally diverted from the criminal justice system by the police; they may be taken directly to mental hospitals or emergency rooms of general hospitals for psychiatric disposition. Here, the police are simply using their discretion in deciding that an individual who has probably committed a crime will be more efficiently and humanely treated outside of the criminal justice system. The elements that go into such decisions are not clear, but limited studies indicate that police respond to the same cues as mental health professionals (Monahan et al. 1979). Offenders who behave in a bizarre manner, seem to be unable to care for themselves, are suicidal, or appear to have limited impulse control are likely to be hospitalized rather than arrested. The nature of the crime and the individual's history of mental illness also play a role in the police officer's decision. Moreover, crimes that fall under the rubric of disorderly conduct are more likely to be seen as manifestations of mental illness. Individuals with previous hospitalizations may be known to the police officer, who may be reluctant to charge them even for a relatively serious crime.

Police officers probably use other cues that are difficult to define. Not infrequently, individuals who have committed identical crimes and have quite similar patterns of mental disorder may be routed to either mental health or correctional systems for reasons that are unclear. This is especially true of alcoholics who commit identical offenses; some of these individuals are repeatedly hospitalized while others are repeatedly jailed.

Certain offenders may be diverted to public or private mental hospitals after the probable-cause hearing or after indictment. This occurs when the court and the prosecution agree that a defendant has some type of emotional disturbance and the defendant is willing to enter a mental hospital. If the crime is not too serious and if the defendant stays in the hospital for several weeks, the charges may be dropped. The same process may be invoked if a defendant agrees to receive psychiatric treatment in an outpatient setting.

A similar type of diversion based on an assumption of mental disorder is available primarily to wealthy defendants. This involves long-term hospitalization in private facilities. As a rule, private institutions that treat long-term patients are very expensive, costing several thousand dollars per month. If wealthy persons commit crimes and seem to be emotionally disturbed, judges and district attorneys may be willing to drop charges against them or delay prosecution if they agree to hospitalization. Much, of course, depends on community sentiment. If the crime is particularly offensive to the community or if it has been extensively publicized, such diversion may not be acceptable irrespective of the defendant's wealth. If, on the other hand, the defendant is viewed sympathetically by the community, the option of long-term hospitalization in a relatively luxurious setting is more likely to be available.

Accurate data on the number of individuals diverted from the criminal justice system to private psychiatric hospitals are almost impossible to obtain. However, from my own work in such hospitals, conversations with others who have worked in similar settings, my work with defendants, and my experience in reviewing insurance claims, I am convinced that the practice is quite common (Halleck 1974). In fact, the number of such individuals is probably much greater than the number who successfully plead insanity.

There is cause to be cynical about this situation. The insanity defense is often referred to as the "rich man's defense." Yet, on a statistical basis, this designation would seem inaccurate, since most insanity acquittees are of lower socioeconomic status (Shah 1986). The real "rich man's defense" for crimes of mild to moderate severity appears to be long-term hospitalization in a private sanatorium.

Characteristics of Formally Adjudicated Mentally Disordered Offenders

Offenders are formally designated as mentally disordered by being found incompetent to proceed in the criminal process, not guilty by reason of insanity, or in need of specialized treatment because they are dangerous or so emotionally disturbed while in prison that they must be transferred to a security hospital. They form a highly diverse group and cannot be classified on the basis of their offenses. They may have been charged with any type of crime,

from first-degree murder to disturbing the peace, although compared with other offenders, a high percentage have committed
crimes of violence. Mentally disordered offenders are also difficult
to classify on the basis of demographic variables, inasmuch as they
include both sexes as well as all socioeconomic classes, races, and
age groups. Caucasians, however, are somewhat overrepresented
when compared with the general prison population (Monahan and
Steadman 1983).

Mentally disordered offenders receive a variety of psychiatric
diagnoses. As a rule, those found incompetent to stand trial are
diagnosed as having a major psychosis. However, some are diagnosed as mentally retarded or have organic brain disorders. Those
found not guilty by reason of insanity are likely to be diagnosed
as psychotic, although some members of this group who have
recovered sufficiently to stand trial may also have severe personality disorders. Generally, inmates transferred from a prison to
a mental hospital are diagnosed as psychotic or as severely
depressed, while some may have secondary diagnoses of personality disorder. Mentally disordered sex offenders or others who
need specialized treatment are most likely to be diagnosed as having personality disorders, although some receive a diagnosis of
mental retardation or psychosis.

The characteristics that formally designated mentally disordered
offenders have in common can be summarized as follows:

1. They are usually diverted from ordinary correctional dispositions and treated in other institutions (viz., security hospitals or
   units). Such diversion can have an important impact upon the
   size of the prison population, since laws and practices that allow for expansion of the number of mentally disordered offenders can help to relieve prison overcrowding. Conversely,
   where diversion is made more difficult, overcrowding may become worse.
2. They are all diagnosed as having a mental disorder that is listed
   in DSM-III, the official manual of the nomenclature of the
   American Psychiatric Association (1980). This means that they
   are likely to have many characteristics in common with those
   ordinarily thought of as mentally ill.
3. They generally require more mental health care and attention
   than ordinary prisoners, and often create difficult administrative problems for institutions where they are kept. If returned
   to traditional custodial settings, they may be a problem to ad-

ministrators insofar as they are viewed as either predators or prey by other prisoners.

4. They tend to be viewed as more dangerous than other offenders. This view is based partially on knowledge of their previous crimes, and partially on a belief that the mental disorder will diminish their responsivity to the ordinary rewards and punishments of the correctional environment or the free world.
5. They are seen as needing some kind of mental health treatment. While the purpose or usefulness of such treatment may be disputed, some effort is usually made to provide it.
6. They are treated by mental health professionals in hospital settings that emphasize security and under conditions similar to those found in prisons.
7. Mentally disordered offenders can generally be committed and restrained in security hospitals under criteria and procedures that are less stringent than regular civil commitment. However, they are released from security hospitals only when they have met criteria and overcome procedures that generally are more stringent.

Where Are Mentally Disordered Offenders Treated?

The institutional placement of formally adjudicated mentally disordered offenders is a complicated matter with important administrative and treatment implications. Most are housed in a hospital setting characterized by a high degree of security. Sometimes a wing or a separate building in a prison is designated a hospital unit for mentally disordered offenders. A wing or separate building of an ordinary mental hospital may be made more secure and similarly designated. In almost half the states, however, offenders are treated in separate institutions specifically built for their care (Kerr and Roth in press). These institutions may be administered by either the mental health or corrections department.

Regardless of where they are located or who is responsible for their administration, the purpose of such institutions is to provide some type of psychiatric treatment in a secure custodial setting. The emphasis on custody predominates, so these institutions are more likely to resemble a prison than a mental hospital. They may be called hospitals for the criminally insane, forensic hospitals, or maximum security hospitals (some criminologists and psychiatrists refer to them unofficially as "hybrid" hospitals). Throughout this monograph the terms "maximum security hospital" or "security hospital" are used to describe either institutions or separate wings or buildings of prisons or public mental hospitals that care for mentally disordered offenders.

The issue of locus of treatment, unfortunately, is even more complicated than the above paragraphs would suggest. Not all formally adjudicated mentally disordered offenders are placed in security hospitals. Those found incompetent to stand trial or not guilty by reason of insanity may be treated at ordinary civil mental hospitals. In most states, women and adolescents are also likely to be housed at civil mental hospitals or in prisons because their numbers do not justify the construction of a special unit. Mentally disordered offenders may also be housed in prisons.

Three other practices confuse the issue of placement even further. First, some prisons contain small units that resemble hospitals and provide brief treatment for mentally disturbed inmates. Inmates sent to these units are not officially transferred and are not formally designated mentally disordered offenders. Second, some states provide separate institutions for different categories of mentally disordered offenders. Those being evaluated for competency may be found in one hospital unit, while transferred prison inmates or sex offenders may be placed in others. Incompetent defendants may be under the jurisdiction of a division of mental health, while sex offenders may be under the jurisdiction of a division of corrections. Third, most security hospitals accept unmanageable patients from civil mental hospitals in their own state. These patients have not been charged with a crime and are not criminal offenders. They are usually violent, however, and are treated with controls as stringent as for the rest of the population.

While further discussion of mentally disordered offenders focuses primarily on those confined and treated in security hospitals, it is important to understand that they may also be treated in other settings. Also, security hospitals differ appreciably from one another in terms of organization, their administrative organizational location (for example, whether they are under a division of mental health, corrections, or another state agency), the manner in which they are administered, the nature of their clientele, and the degree of their commitment to a treatment model. The major quality they share is a heavy emphasis on custody.

Attitudes Toward Mentally Disordered Offenders

Those formally designated as mentally disordered offenders on the basis of some judicial or administrative process tend to be treated inconsistently by our society. We view them as both "mad" and "bad," and over time we tend to emphasize one of these attributions more than the other in determining how to deal with them. Sometimes mentally disordered offenders are treated more harshly than ordinary offenders; sometimes their treatment is more benevolent. Insofar as they do not fit clearly into either the mental health or correctional model of treatment, these individuals tend to pose difficult management problems for most institutions.

In 1857 the American psychiatrist Edward Jarvis wrote the following eloquent words in describing the plight of mentally disordered offenders:

> But the insane criminal has nowhere any home: no age or nation has provided a place for him. He is everywhere unwelcome and objectionable. The prisons thrust him out; the hospitals are unwilling to receive him; the law will not let him stay at his house, and the public will not permit him to go abroad. And yet humanity and justice, the sense of common danger, and a tender regard for a deeply degraded brother-man, all agree that something should be done for him . . . . (Jarvis 1857, as quoted in American Psychiatric Association 1984, pp. 192-193)

These words still apply to mentally disordered offenders today. We remain uncertain how to treat them. We are unwilling to leave them alone, yet most agencies seek to avoid responsibility for their care. We confine them to prisons and to prison-like hospitals where they are sometimes treated worse than other offenders. They almost always receive worse treatment than mental patients in public or private mental hospitals.

Although our society does not invest a great deal of money or energy in their day-to-day management, mentally disordered offenders are hardly ignored by those concerned with the moral and legal issues of punishment and treatment. Among these groups, mentally disordered offenders have few friends. Many concerned citizens have an exaggerated view of the dangerousness of mentally disordered offenders and a distorted impression that they are treated with exceptional gentleness by the criminal justice system. Given the prevalence of this view, public figures who can project an image of being "tough on crime" or who argue that mentally disordered offenders are "beating the rap" can gain a certain political advantage. Too often, the media and ambitious politicians tend to seek out the "tough position" on management of mentally disordered offenders. Public misconceptions may be strengthened by recounting "atrocity" stories that usually involve a detailed description of a crime committed by a mentally disordered offender released from a hospital after only a brief period of confinement. Unfortunately, public figures gain less attention or support when they present these issues in a more temperate manner.

The main friends of mentally disordered offenders are those responsible for their day-to-day care and certain legal groups who have sought to expand their rights. Correctional officials and mental health professionals struggle to help the mentally disordered offender in spite of being handicapped by inadequate resources. Since these caretakers are obligated to exert control over offenders to protect the public, offenders do not always appreciate their efforts. Nevertheless, many who work directly with mentally disordered offenders retain a remarkably strong commitment to helping them.

Civil liberties attorneys have in the past two decades devoted considerable efforts to protecting the rights of offenders. Through litigation or related efforts, they have sought to protect the procedural rights of mentally disordered offenders and to improve their conditions of incarceration and treatment. While they have had some notable successes, their effectiveness in bringing about major changes is uncertain (Ennis and Embry 1978).

Academicians who study mentally disordered offenders could conceivably use their conclusions to support better treatment. Actually, academic views of crime and punishment have been used to support both compassionate and retributive approaches. During eras when society demands greater control of deviant behavior, a scholarly theory that can be interpreted as supporting a harsher correctional approach may be used to justify repressive practices irrespective of the intentions of its author. The "just deserts" model, for example, was resurrected in the 1970s as a fair and humane way of imposing punishment (Morris 1974). In the hands of some legislatures it has, unfortunately, become a rationale for imposing unusually lengthy sentences.

As an academician interested in criminology and criminal law for the past 30 years, but with a background as a clinician and correctional administrator, I approach the problems of the mentally disordered offender with no pretense of neutrality. My views can be summarized as follows.

The mentally disordered offender cannot be understood without considering the total system of criminal justice. I believe that the current criminal justice practices that focus so heavily on lengthy imprisonment of all types of offenders are shamefully severe and very expensive. This severity creates so much concern with the individual rights of offenders that an enormous degree of litigation is promoted, which does not further the need of society. Can a system of criminal justice that focuses steadfastly on a philosophy of retribution and deals primarily with the nature of the crime rather than the nature of the criminal provide maximum protection for the public? All the procedures and practices by which we identify and treat mentally disordered offenders can be viewed as costly efforts to preserve a system that does not work well. A return to the almost abandoned restraint/rehabilitation model of criminal justice should be seriously considered.

My views certainly do not flow with the current tide of opinion. It is especially important, therefore, that the reader be aware of them as the theoretical and practical issues raised by mentally disordered offenders are discussed.

CHAPTER 2

Societal Responses
to Social Deviance

THE POLICIES THAT DETERMINE the disposition and treatment of mentally disordered offenders are derived from broader societal policies dealing with the general problem of criminal conduct. Society's response to crime is determined by three sometimes conflicting objectives: promotion of justice, protection of the public, and beneficence.

Justice

While doing justice is an obvious purpose of any legally sanctioned response to social conflict or antisocial behavior, justice is extremely difficult to define. As generally used, the term refers to equitableness and rightness (Rawls 1971). In a statement attributed to Socrates in the first book of the Republic, justice was defined simply as "giving to each man what is proper for him." Criminal justice is usually concerned with the proper degree of punishment to impose on an offender.

The guiding principle of punishment in Anglo-Saxon law has been that of "desert" (Hart 1968). We impose harm upon offenders in direct proportion to the harm we believe they have inflicted upon society. In so doing we express society's moral condemnation. The concept of "just deserts," in addition to expressing society's wish to retaliate, also limits the degree of punishment that can be inflicted upon offenders. Morris notes that the concept of "deserts" limits sanctions to no more than those "deserved" by the crime (Morris 1982).

Justice also implies fair or equitable treatment of offenders. One aspect of fairness requires offenders who have inflicted the same harm upon society under similar circumstances to be treated in similar fashion, i.e., equally. This notion of fairness predominates in our criminal justice system where punishment is usually designed to fit the crime, not the criminal. Another aspect of fairness that is considered less frequently relates to differences among offenders. Treating two offenders who have committed the same act in exactly the same way may not be fair if the offenders actually have different capacities to control their behavior, to defend themselves in the criminal process, or to be influenced by punishment or treatment. Sometimes the interest of justice is best served by treating individuals who have imposed similar harms upon society differently, i.e., unequally.

Protecting the Public

While justice in the sense of "deserts" is currently viewed as a major guiding moral principle of our criminal justice system, the degree of punishment imposed upon offenders is also determined by a more utilitarian purpose of the law, viz., protecting society. Protection of the public, like "deserts," often justifies punishment. Two traditional arguments support this retributive stance:

1. Punishing offenders may deter them from committing subsequent crimes (specific or special deterrence). It also firmly reminds others that crime will be followed by punishment, thereby inhibiting illegal acts (general deterrence). Even if *fear* of punishment were not a deterrent, the public pronouncement of punishment might still deter others by teaching them in a dramatic way the existing social rules.
2. If the state punishes offenders it will diminish the likelihood of private vengeance. The assumption here is that if the state does not punish offenders, the victims of crime or their loved ones would.

A less traditional but nevertheless utilitarian argument for retribution is that punishment "adds bite" to the ascription of responsibility placed upon offenders. Punishment is a powerful reminder of blameworthiness, and the rest of society is dramatically informed and reminded about prohibited behaviors. Punishment will, it is hoped, cause offenders to accept responsibility for their illegal acts and assume greater responsibility for their subsequent actions. They will be more receptive to societal demands for appropriate behavior, and they may be better subjects of rehabilitation.

There is some affinity between the goals of seeking justice by doing to offenders what they deserve and protecting society by using punishment as a deterrent. Both goals emphasize providing degrees of punishment based on the severity of the crimes rather than on the personal characteristics of the offender. Both goals encourage the use of punishment, such as imprisonment, that can be quantified so as to inflict the precise amount necessary to promote justice or public safety. While advocates of the "deserts" model are not always concerned with the utilitarian purpose of deterrence, in practice society tends to rely on principles of both deserts and deterrence when it imprisons people. To the extent that these principles are combined, they can be conceived as constituting one of the major models of the criminal justice system, subsequently referred to herein as the desert/deterrence model. The penalties justified by this model are referred to as retributive justice.

The goal of protecting the public may also support nonretributive interventions. People may be subjected to physical (or sometimes chemical) restraints or incapacitation simply to prevent them from harming others. When restraint is invoked primarily to protect the public, no punishment may be intended. Societal protection may also be the major motivation in efforts to rehabilitate offenders. To the extent that individuals who might continue to commit crimes are somehow influenced to refrain from doing so in the future, the public will obviously receive greater protection.

Beneficence

Society's beneficent motivations toward deviant individuals are usually expressed in terms of providing rehabilitation and treatment, of protecting individual rights, or of granting mercy. Actually, we attempt to rehabilitate offenders for two main reasons: we believe their reformation assures more protection for society, and we believe that those who want to lead a law-abiding life achieve more happiness. When rehabilitation is emphasized for the purpose of helping the offender, the societal objective may be viewed as beneficent.

Beneficence is only one of society's objectives in protecting the rights of deviant individuals. The practical reasons for wanting to afford such protection include an awareness that by protecting the rights of those who are currently viewed as deviant, we ultimately protect ourselves. Even such a practical concern with individual rights, however, is based on at least some degree of beneficence insofar as it requires an effort to empathize or identify with the potential suffering of other persons.

Finally, beneficence may mitigate the retribution imposed upon offenders. The criminal law often identifies certain characteristics of offenders (such as previous contributions to the society or various psychological or social incapacities) that justify giving them a lesser sentence. At times the courts may even be merciful toward those who have done great harm to society. The quality of mercy may also be evident in efforts to minimize the oppressive aspects of incarceration. When correctional practices are based on a belief that loss of liberty is sufficient punishment, efforts may be made to keep prison conditions from becoming so oppressive that they impose an additional burden upon the offender (Sykes 1958). Beneficence may have only an ephemeral influence on the criminal justice system, but its influence nevertheless exists.

The goal of protecting the public may sometimes be combined with the goal of beneficence in establishing a restraint/rehabilitation model of criminal justice. Under this model, efforts are made to rehabilitate offenders who are likely to be restrained until rehabilitation is accomplished. Restraint/rehabilitation models are consistent with beneficent motivations when rehabilitation is intended to help the offender.

Treatment of the Non-Criminal Mentally Ill and Mentally Disordered Offenders

Some of the problems created by mentally disordered offenders may be better understood by considering the motivations that govern society's different responses to the mentally ill and to offenders. With the mentally ill, society is guided primarily by the values of protecting the public and of beneficence toward the afflicted. It invokes a restraint/rehabilitation model to achieve this goal. Patients are only restrained to protect them or others until they have been rehabilitated. While patients may experience restraint as punitive, and while it may in fact be harmful to them, punishment is not intended. The issue of retribution does not arise unless a mentally disordered person commits an act that is defined as a crime. The mentally ill can be quite disruptive to society; they may have psychotic outbursts on the street, be publicly intoxicated, or behave in a variety of annoying and bizarre ways.

But as long as their behavior is not defined as criminal, society has no desire to punish them.

With ordinary offenders, society seeks to provide justice, protect itself, and be benevolent at the same time. When a person accused of committing a crime is also believed to be mentally disordered, the needs for justice, beneficence, and public protection are especially difficult to balance.

If an offender is believed to be incapacitated at the time of the crime or becomes incapacitated any time in the process of trial or imprisonment, the quest for fairness and beneficence may limit the severity of retribution based on the notion of desert. The existence of mental illness also leads society to question the deterrent value of punishment. We sometimes doubt that the seriously mentally ill learn from punishment or that punishing them is really necessary to deter others. Once the utilitarian aspect of punishing mentally disordered offenders is questioned, we may seek other ways of dealing with them. If they do not seem dangerous, we may put them on probation or allow them to seek treatment in public or private mental health facilities. The primary motivation here is beneficent. If we perceive mentally ill offenders as dangerous, however, we may put them in specialized programs where they are restrained and treated for the purpose of rehabilitation. The primary motivation here is societal protection, but elements of beneficence may also be involved.

Methods for handling mentally disordered offenders change as society's commitment to the values of justice, societal protection, and beneficence changes. Society's responses to the socially deviant are not fixed. Even within as short a period as a decade, the balance among these values may shift dramatically. Such shifts have a powerful impact upon the policies and processes by which mentally disordered offenders are formally identified and diverted from the criminal justice system.

CHAPTER 3

Lack of Capacity to Proceed
in the Criminal Justice Process

IN DEALING WITH ALL OFFENDERS, society must balance its need to dispense justice and protect the public with its beneficent concern for the rights of accused individuals. This balancing process leads to the development of rules and procedures that provide certain protections and impose certain restraints upon offenders as they move through the criminal justice process. This chapter focuses on defendants who have been indicted but whose mental incapacities are believed to be such that the fairness of subjecting them to the criminal justice process is questionable.

Incompetent Offenders

The Rationale for Diversion

In an adversary system of justice, persons charged with a crime must be given an adequate opportunity to defend themselves. Sometimes they cannot do so because they are incapacitated by a mental disorder or other disability. Defendants who are compromised in their ability to recall events, produce evidence, weigh various options, or accurately perceive or understand the many situations they encounter following arrest and indictment may be substantially handicapped in their ability to enter a plea or to participate in plea bargaining. In addition, their ability to testify in their defense, confront witnesses, or project a suitable demeanor to the judge and jury may impair their capacity to defend themselves in the courtroom. Although most criminals avoid trial through plea bargaining, the competence of defendants to enter a plea or to plea bargain is rarely considered in the criminal justice system. Most often the question of capacity to proceed is framed in terms of the competency of defendants to stand trial.

The doctrine of pretrial incompetency has common law origins going back to mid-17th century England (Group for the Advancement of Psychiatry 1974). In the early 1900s, the U.S. Supreme Court recognized a constitutional basis for postponing criminal proceedings against those believed to be incompetent (Wilnick 1983). In the past decade, the court affirmed the incompetency plea and characterized the prohibition against trying an incompetent defendant as "fundamental to an adversary system of justice" (*Drope v. Missouri* 1975).

The incompetency doctrine is believed to protect the integrity of the criminal proceeding by promoting the accuracy, fairness, and dignity of the trial process (Brakel and Rock 1971). If defendants could not provide their attorneys with the information required for an effective defense, the level of fact-finding accuracy in the trial process would be diminished. Neither society nor the individual could be sure that all the major issues were fairly considered in the course of adjudication. Trials of individuals incapable of assisting in their own defense would also make the verdict of guilty less significant as a symbol of justice. Some in society might be concerned that if the defendant had been fully competent the outcome would have been different. It can even be argued that without the incompetency doctrine, all guilty verdicts would have less impact upon society because there would always be some concern that they were reached through unfair proceedings. Finally, if incompetent defendants were tried, the integrity and dignity of the legal process could be jeopardized. Trying individuals who may not even understand why they are on trial is inherently absurd, as well as incompatible with the commitment to justice. The decorum of the court may also suffer when a defendant behaves bizarrely or remains mute and uncomprehending throughout the proceedings.

Initiating Evaluations of Competency

A request for determination of competency usually is made at the time of arraignment, but it could be made at any subsequent point in the criminal justice process. Not infrequently, the issue is first raised during the trial. On rare occasions, persons who have been found guilty have subsequently become mentally ill and been found incompetent to be sentenced (*Wojtowicz v. United States*

1977). Offenders can even be found incompetent to be executed. The rationale may be based on protecting the defendant's right of appeal, but it is also related to notions of justice and retribution. Offenders must know why they are being punished and must be able to seek forgiveness.

The request for competency evaluation is usually based on observations by police officers, jail officials, family, or participating attorneys that the defendant is behaving strangely and appears to be emotionally disturbed. Sometimes the request is determined by the nature of the crime. If a crime is bizarre, and particularly if it receives a great deal of publicity, a request for pretrial competency determination is very likely. Prosecution for certain crimes, such as attempting to harm the President of the United States, almost assures that such a request will be made.

The request may be made by defense attorneys, prosecutors, or judges. In addition to their concern with accuracy, fairness, and dignity, each group may have special reasons for wanting the defendant's competency assessed. Defense attorneys may wish to delay the trial. With the passage of time, witnesses against the defendant may lose interest in testifying or be unavailable for other reasons. Defense attorneys may wish to have their clients examined by a psychiatrist for other legal purposes. This may be especially critical when the client is indigent, since the cost of the evaluation is assumed by the court or by public mental health facilities (e.g., forensic clinics or security hospitals). The psychiatrist's report can be used to determine whether a plea of not guilty by reason of insanity might be considered. Mitigating factors relating to mental impairment may also be discovered and introduced at the time of sentencing.

Defense attorneys may also seek more information about the psychological state of their clients in order to defend them more effectively. Most attorneys believe they can provide a better defense if they are aware of their clients' psychological strengths and deficiencies. Finally, some defense attorneys probably view the incompetency plea as a means of helping their clients "beat the rap." They hope that once found incompetent their clients will be civilly committed or released or at least "do easier time" in a security hospital than in a prison (Steadman 1979).

Prosecutors may ask for a competency examination to avoid having the conviction overruled on appeal. They have also been known to invoke competency proceedings over the defendant's objection in order to avoid a criminal trial when the state's evidence was weak. Defendants who are found incompetent to stand trial commonly spend weeks or even months in a maximum security hospital. (Although the type of hospital or prison unit to which a mentally disordered offender is sent varies from state to state, these units are consistently more security and punishment oriented than ordinary mental hospitals). The prosecutor then obtains one of the results of a criminal conviction, viz., confinement, without struggling through a trial in which the defendant would have substantial procedural protection (such as the right to a trial by jury and conviction based on proof beyond a reasonable doubt), which might favor acquittal. Finding a defendant incompetent to stand trial is one way prosecutors can ensure that offenders they believe to be dangerously ill will, at least temporarily, be kept off the streets.

Judges may request competency examinations to avoid being overruled on appeal (*Drope v. Missouri* 1975; *Pate v. Robinson* 1966). Some judges also view the examination as a means of obtaining additional psychiatric information about the defendant. The judge may wish to consider this information at the time of sentencing. Or, the judge's motivations may be similar to that of the prosecutor, viz., to ensure some confinement and restraint of allegedly dangerous offenders pending their trial. Sometimes judges as well as other legal functionaries are tempted to send "nuisance" cases (i.e., defendants charged with minor crimes who are obviously mentally ill, but who do not meet the requirements for civil commitment) for competency evaluation. Judges have also been accused of invoking the competency examination to spare the community the chore of dealing with the troubling moral or political issues raised by certain cases (Szasz 1972). For example, if a prominent figure committed a criminal act against the state, a trial would serve to legitimate the dissent but a finding of incompetency would raise the possibility that the act was irrational rather than motivated by political or moral considerations.

The Evaluation Process

The competency examination is usually performed by psychiatrists, although in many jurisdictions examinations by clinical psychologists are also accepted. The offender is examined either in the community or at a more distant hospital. If community evaluation is allowed, it may be conducted on an outpatient basis in a doctor's office, at a community mental health center, or even in a private hospital. More frequently, when the defendant is not able to meet bail, it is performed in the local jail or a security hospital. Examinations performed in the community tend to be reported fairly promptly to the court, usually in a few days. Although the trend is toward evaluating defendants in their own communities, most competency examinations are probably still conducted in security hospitals or units set aside for the assessment and treatment of mentally disordered offenders. This is most likely to happen when the defendant has been charged with a serious crime, especially a crime of violence. One study estimated that 25,000 defendants were evaluated for competency to stand trial in special mental health or correctional facilities in 1978 (Steadman and Hartstone 1983). Defendants sent to maximum security institutions may be restrained for several weeks or even months while the evaluation is conducted. During that time they are denied bail and the opportunity to plea bargain. Critics of the incompetency diversion note that during this time defendants may be seriously compromised in their ability to assist in locating witnesses or in other aspects of preparing their cases (Halpern 1975).

While the majority of defendants are examined only by state-employed mental health professionals who presumably have no interest in whether the defendant is punished, defendants with sufficient financial means can also hire their own experts. Presumably, mental health clinicians employed by defendants will testify in support of their clients' interests. Some defendants, particularly those charged with serious crimes that they know they have committed, may welcome the incompetency diversion. Delays in the trial may favor their acquittal, and being found incompetent may encourage the court to be more lenient if they are ultimately convicted and sentenced (Roesch and Golding 1979). These defendants may have good reason to hire their own experts to testify as to their competency. Other defendants, particularly those charged with minor crimes, may not wish to be found incompetent. They may not welcome delays in their trials, or they may wish to plea bargain. Their concern is that they could be institutionalized longer if found incompetent than if tried and convicted. If the request for competency examination is made by the prosecution or the court, these individuals might seek their own experts to testify that they are competent to proceed. Occasionally, prosecutors hire mental health clinicians as expert witnesses. This almost always occurs when they want a defendant who is charged with a serious crime to be found competent to stand trial.

When all examinations are completed, defendants return to court where the judge reviews the psychiatric reports and determines their competency to proceed. In most instances, defendants are examined by only one psychiatrist, and with rare exceptions the court accepts the recommendation made by that state-employed expert. Competency hearings are usually brief and nonadversarial. In most cases defendants are found competent and their trials proceed. If defendants are found incompetent, however, their trials are again delayed as the state assumes the obligation of restoring their competence. Some defendants found incompetent may be allowed to undergo outpatient treatment. Frequently, however, they are sent to an institution for mentally disordered offenders (often the same one that examined them) where various treatments are used to restore their competency.

From this point on, several dispositions are possible. The most common outcome is that competency is restored and defendants are returned to court to stand trial. If competency is not restored, defendants may remain for several months at a security hospital, or they may be committed to an ordinary mental hospital that treats other civilly committed patients.

Although most defendants who are evaluated for competency are found competent and are quickly returned to court, a substantial number are not. According to one survey, 6,420 were admitted to mental health or correctional institutions as incompetent to stand trial in 1978 (Steadman and Hartstone 1983). No data are available on the number adjudicated incompetent in that year but not institutionalized. Those adjudicated incompetent and also institutionalized comprised 32 percent of all admissions to hospitals or prison units dealing with mentally disordered offenders in 1978. In the same year, 3,400 persons found incompetent to stand trial were residing in these institutions. (The number of residents on a given day is less than the number of yearly admissions, since most of these people are institutionalized for less than a year.) The pretrial incompetents constituted 17 percent of the institutionalized mentally disordered offender population in 1978 (Steadman and Hartstone, 1983).

Disposition of Defendants Who Do Not Regain Competency

Prior to 1973, no constitutional limits were placed on how long incompetent defenders could be kept in maximum security institutions; often they faced long and indeterminate confinement. In 1972, the Supreme Court limited the time that pretrial incompetent persons could be retained in maximum security hospital units specifically set aside for mentally disordered offenders. The Court ruled:

We hold, consequently, that a person charged by a state with a criminal offense who is committed solely on account of his incapacity to proceed to trial cannot be held more than the reasonable period of time necessary to determine whether there is a substantial probability that he will attain that capacity in the foreseeable future. If it is determined that this is not the case, then the state must either institute the customary civil commitment proceeding that would be required to commit indefinitely any other citizen, or release the defendant. Furthermore, even if it is determined that the defendant probably soon will be able to stand trial, his continued commitment must be justified by progress toward that goal. (*Jackson v. Indiana* 1972, p.738)

A number of states have attempted to implement the Supreme Court's decision and now require patients who have been found incompetent and are not progressing toward restoration of their competency to be either civilly committed or released. Some states also require the criminal charges to be dropped when the defendants' time in an institution equals the time they would have served if convicted (Wilnick and Demo 1980).

The Supreme Court ruling does not completely resolve the problem of what to do with those defendants who are unlikely to regain competency, the so-called "unrestorable" incompetents (Morris 1983). Sometimes neither civil commitment nor outright release is a satisfactory solution. Some of these persons cannot be committed because they do not meet the mental illness requirement of most civil commitment statutes. (Their incompetence may stem from a handicap such as deafness, mutism, or severe mental retardation, and they may have no recognizable mental illness.) In theory, even defendants charged with violent acts may not meet the dangerousness requirement of many civil commitment statutes. Incompetent defendants have, after all, not been tried and their violence has not been proven. Under current commitment standards, "unrestorable" incompetents who have actually committed violent crimes might be released. In some states, fear of this possibility has encouraged legislation that allows for continued retention of incompetents believed to be dangerous who do not meet the criteria for civil commitment (Morris 1983). Such legislation tends to subvert the Supreme Court's decision in *Jackson*.

While "unrestorable" incompetents are few in number, their ultimate disposition is a matter of considerable concern to society. One case received national attention, that of Donald Lang, an illiterate deaf mute who was twice arrested and charged with murder. Because he did not meet the requirements of either competency to stand trial or civil commitment (he was not found to be mentally ill), and since he was viewed as a highly dangerous person, the courts could not find a humane disposition for this man that also protected the public (*Illinois v. Lang* 1979). In this type of situation it is almost impossible simultaneously to protect the rights of defendants and those of the public. The fear that dangerous defendants will be released or that nondangerous defendants will be indeterminately confined has fueled the arguments of some legal scholars who urge that the incompetency plea should be drastically modified or even abolished (Burt and Morris 1972; Halpern 1975).

Competency to Proceed: The Legal Criteria

Although jurisdictions vary in the exact definition of competency to stand trial, all statutes deal with the defendant's fitness to understand the charges against him, to understand the judicial process, and to rationally cooperate with an attorney in his own defense. These criteria are derived from the Supreme Court's decision in *Dusky v. United States* (1960), in which the Court ruled that it is not sufficient that

> the defendant is oriented to time and place and has some recollection of events, [but rather] whether he has sufficient present ability to consult with his lawyer with a reasonable degree of rational understanding and whether he has a rational as well as factual understanding of the proceeding against him.

This standard requires the assessment of both cognitive and communicative skills. In some jurisdictions, the lack of these skills must be specifically related to a mental illness. The *Dusky* standard, however, does not require that mental illness be the only basis for incompetency to stand trial. Defendants who are unable to communicate with their attorney for whatever reason (e.g., deafness or mutism) might also be found incompetent.

A federal court decision spelled out in specific detail the cognitive and communicative skills required for determining a defendant's pretrial competency. The opinion stated:

(1) that he has mental capacity to appreciate his presence in relation to time, place and things;

(2) that his elementary mental processes be such that he ap-

prehends (i.e., seizes and grasps with what mind he has) that he is in a Court of Justice, charged with a criminal offense;

(3) that there is a Judge on the Bench;

(4) a Prosecutor is present who will try to convict him on a criminal charge;

(5) that he has a lawyer (self-employed or Court-appointed) who will undertake to defend him against that charge;

(6) that he will be expected to tell his lawyer the circumstances, to the best of his mental ability (whether colored or not by mental aberration), the facts surrounding him at the time and place where the law violation is alleged to have been committed;

(7) that there is, or will be, a jury present to pass upon evidence adduced as to his guilt or innocence of such charge; and

(8) he has memory sufficient to relate those things in his own personal manner. (*Wieter v. Settle* 1961, pp. 321-322)

Problems of Mental Health Evaluations

Some controversy has arisen over how mental health professionals should evaluate pretrial competency. In most jurisdictions, the evaluating clinicians are not required to describe the basis of their conclusions. They simply testify that the defendant is incompetent to proceed according to the particular standard used in their jurisdiction. In past years, and occasionally even today, psychiatrists and other clinicians tend to equate incompetency with psychosis or severe mental illness (Ennis 1972), ignoring the reality that such individuals might nevertheless be effective defendants. The modern trend is to find incompetency only when specific and legally relevant incapacities are apparent (Robey 1965). Checklists are used to help clinicians consider specific issues, such as the defendant's ability to relate to attorneys, to plan legal strategy, and to understand court procedures as well as the range and nature of possible penalties. Some of these checklists are quite detailed (McGarry et al. 1973). Their growing popularity has added consistency to clinical reporting. They have played an important role in helping mental health professionals focus on the real issues of competency and have probably contributed to a decrease in the percentage of examined defendants who are found incompetent.

The role of attorneys in competency assessments is currently quite limited. Only rarely are they consulted with regard to the first element of the *Dusky* standard, viz., whether the defendant "has sufficient present ability to consult with his lawyer with a reasonable degree of rational understanding." It is difficult to understand why lawyers are left out of the evaluation process, since they may be in the best position to evaluate the defendant's ability to provide them with the kind of information needed for an adequate defense. Attorneys could also help in assessing the level of functioning required for a particular case. The adequacy of a defendant's capabilities would be expected to vary with the attorney's plans regarding such issues as the number of witnesses to be called, whether to plea bargain, and whether to put the defendant on the stand.

Even with extremely thorough evaluations based on precise criteria for competency, the accuracy of many competency evaluations may still be questionable. Competency to perform a particular task, such as effectively assisting in one's own defense, is not easily defined. The competency of defendants will vary with the degree of stress imposed upon them at any given moment and by even minor fluctuations in their mental statuses. The experience and skill of the defense attorney is yet another highly relevant factor. Evaluators, at best, can only predict how defendants are likely to perform in court. This prediction must be made without precise knowledge of how stressful the trial will actually be. It must also be based on the evaluation of the mental status of defendants at the time they are examined, which may be weeks or months before the trial takes place. By the time defendants are actually tried, their mental condition may have appreciably changed.

The inherent difficulties in assessing competency to stand trial are complicated even further when defendants are evaluated in hospitals where they are simultaneously treated. Hospital environments bear little resemblance to courtrooms. Some defendants become more disturbed and seem less competent in response to the hospital setting. They may be denied the opportunity to proceed in the criminal justice process when they may actually be capable of defending themselves. A more common response is for the defendant to become more subdued and thus appear more competent in the hospital, particularly if pharmacological treatment is provided. However, there is really no way of knowing how well defendants retain their new-found tranquility when they return to the trial process. Many are returned to jails where they are exposed to high levels of stress. There may also be no way of knowing if they receive or actually take their prescribed medicine. By the time they reach the courtroom, they may have quite different capacities than they had at the time of their evaluation.

Legal Issues

The Influence of Societal Values on Current Practices

The diversion of defendants who lack capacity to proceed in the criminal justice process is influenced by society's emphasis on retributive justice. To the extent that a society is committed to imposing severe penalties on offenders but also wishes to be fair and benevolent, extraordinary pains must be taken to ensure the guilt of those who are punished. This in turn requires that individuals subjected to the criminal justice process receive every conceivable protection from undeserved or unfair punishment. In the last two decades, when society's commitment to retributive justice has been high, requests for incompetency evaluations have also increased. When the stakes are high, criminal justice proceedings become more adversarial and our sense of fairness prompts concerns that a defendant not be allowed to enter the ordeal of legal combat with a handicap. It should be clear, however, that society's benevolence in this situation arises as a consequence of its initial wish for retribution.

Once individuals are found incompetent to proceed in the criminal process and are diverted, society must deal with the issue of self-protection. If those diverted are believed to be dangerous, then it is in the public interest to restrain them until they can be returned to court or, if this is not possible, until they can be treated and safely released.

The incompetency issue highlights the extent to which an excessive societal commitment to the retributive aspect of justice can lead to convoluted and sometimes even absurd criminal justice practices. I have noted that occasionally offenders may be found incompetent to be sentenced. The most macabre example occurs when our legal system becomes concerned with an person's competency to be executed, believing that it is unjust to execute individuals who do not know why they are being killed or who cannot rationally seek forgiveness at the last minute (Slovenko 1973). More common examples arise when a society, preoccupied with retributive justice, also becomes concerned with creating procedural protections that are fair to psychologically impaired offenders. Recently, a number of proposals have been made for going forward with the trials of those whose competency cannot be restored (Burt and Morris 1972; Morris 1982; Halpern 1975). These require significant changes in various aspects of the trial procedure, including changes in rules of evidence, instructions to the jury, and the defendant's right of appeal. The suggested changes are efforts to compensate for incapacities of defendants by lightening their procedural burdens and by imposing procedural handicaps upon the state. These suggestions, which make some sense as a solution to problems created by an emphasis on retributive justice, also illustrate the extent to which the criminal trial can approximate a sporting event in which the rules must be periodically changed to keep both sides competitive.

Does the Incompetency Diversion Serve the Interest of Justice?

In assessing the extent to which the incompetency diversion meets the societal objective of justice, most commentators focus either on the possibility that some defendants will try to be found incompetent to avoid—or at least delay—punishment, or that others who may be innocent, or guilty only of minor crimes, will have the incompetency diversion thrust upon them and serve excessive lengths of time in mental institutions (Scull 1977; Ennis and Hansen 1976). The fear that a significant number of incompetent defendants will "beat the rap" is probably unfounded. Recent research in this area indicates that defendants found incompetent tend to be confined as long as those tried and convicted of similar offenses (Steadman 1979). The *Jackson* decision could, in theory, change this situation (*Jackson v. Indiana* 1972). Conceivably, a large number of "unrestorable incompetents" who fail to meet the criteria of civil commitment might simply be allowed to go free. But thus far, there is little evidence that this is happening (Morris 1982).

The possibility that the incompetency diversion will compromise the civil rights of defendants must be taken more seriously. One concern is that defendants will be held in security hospitals indefinitely. In the pre-*Jackson* era many defendants charged with minor crimes were incarcerated for years without being tried (Hess 1961; McGarry et al. 1973). In those days, defendants found incompetent were at significant risk of spending more time in security hospitals than they would have spent in prison if tried, found guilty, and incarcerated (McGarry and Bendt 1969). Since the *Jackson* decision, however, it appears that unusually lengthy confinement in security hospitals is diminishing (Roesch and Golding 1980). Even where the implementation of the *Jackson* standards has moved slowly, the amount of time incompetent defendants spend hospitalized remains quite similar to the time they would have spent in prison (Steadman and Hartstone 1983).

Another civil liberty concern relates to the disadvantages that defendants suffer while confined to security hospitals for restoration of their competency. The loss of opportunity for bail and plea bargaining has already been noted. Additional risks include the possibility that the defendant is innocent and may be deprived of a chance to prove it, or that evidence favoring the defendant's case might be lost. The latter event might impair the prosecutor's case as well. Such adverse consequences bolster the arguments of those who favor the abolition or substantial modification of the incompetency plea (Burt and Morris 1972; Halpern 1975).

Another Issue of Fairness

The incompetency plea raises another issue of fairness within the criminal justice system that is rarely considered. If all defendants have the right to mount an adequate defense, then the issue of competency should be raised much more frequently. A large number of defendants have psychological and social handicaps that substantially limit their capacity to participate or cooperate in their own defense. The criminal justice system might achieve a greater degree of fairness if it regularly considered the capacity of these individuals to proceed. (It should be clear that in making this argument, I am not implying that unjust convictions are frequent. Since the great majority of defendants who are convicted are probably guilty, any lack of competence during their criminal proceedings may not be of major significance. I also recognize that in many criminal trial proceedings, defendants are not required to do very much and may be adequately defended even though they lack many of the attributes usually associated with competency.)

The capacity to proceed in the criminal process is distributed along a continuum; it is not an absolute either/or quality. No two offenders have exactly the same capacity to defend themselves at trial. Some defendants have exceptionally good capacities and others exceptionally bad. Those who are blessed with superior financial or psychological capacities will have a better chance to avoid punishment than those who are not. Any legal standard of incompetency must exclude some individuals whose level of incapacity is severe, but just above the threshold set by that standard. The likelihood that the excluded group, who are substantially impaired, is very large can be illustrated by considering the psychological qualities required of hypothetically optimal or "perfect" defendants.

1. Perfect defendants should have excellent memories. They need to remember as much as possible about their whereabouts at the time of the offense and all details about witnesses or parties involved in the proceedings. Memory is just one aspect of intelligence that is useful. Brighter defendants can be expected to respond more quickly and effectively as witnesses in their own behalf. They will also be more helpful in planning their defense and assisting their counsel in the cross-examination of witnesses.

Attorneys who work regularly with criminal defendants probably have the best sense of how incapacitated many of them are. Public defenders who deal with the indigent very quickly become aware of the ineptitude of their clients. Many defendants have severe cognitive deficits. Only rarely do they accurately recall details regarding the crime, their whereabouts, or the whereabouts of witnesses. But poor memories are not related only to limited intelligence or self-serving motivations. A substantial number of offenders were intoxicated at the time of the crime, and their defective memory may be a genuine product of temporary brain dysfunction. Moreover, most defendants fail to appreciate the subtle nuances of the law or the trial process. With the exception of "battle-hardened" chronic offenders, they are neither articulate witnesses nor keen observers of legal proceedings.

2. Perfect defendants need to sustain functional levels of anxiety during the pretrial phase. Too little anxiety is undesirable. They need to remain tense enough to perceive as many visual and auditory stimuli as possible. They need to be alert enough to relate courtroom stimuli to past learning and to understand their significance. On the other hand, too much anxiety might immobilize them. Even a moderate degree of anxiety might preclude their maintaining sufficient concentration to respond to significant cues or to make rational judgments.

No defendant is likely to approach a criminal proceeding with an optimal level of anxiety. This is especially true in the phase of criminal proceedings where most cases are settled, namely, before trial where a plea may be negotiated. The question of the competency of a defendant to plea bargain has received little attention in the criminal justice literature, yet close to 90 percent of criminal adjudications involve plea negotiations and critical decisions about pleading guilty (Silberman 1978). The decision to plead guilty has profound ramifications for the defendant. One court has held that competency to make such a decision should require even more demanding criteria than those used to assess competency to stand trial (*Sieling v. Syman* 1973). It is precisely at this stage of the criminal justice proceedings, however, that defendants are most psychologically vulnerable. Those familiar with conditions in most American jails appreciate that defendants who have spent weeks or months under conditions of substantial deprivation and at high risk of being assaulted or raped, are limited in their ability to approach the issue of plea bargaining rationally. Many live in a state of constant fear, manifested by difficulty in thinking and psychic numbness. At this stage of the proceedings, jailed defendants can be influenced by threats or promises that would have little effect on a normal person.

Our society does not usually expect as much from others who have been severely traumatized. It is interesting to compare society's concern about the psychological impact of being a prisoner of war or a hostage with its concern about the psychological impact of being a jailed defendant. These two predicaments differ in many ways but they also have some interesting similarities. Both groups experience physical and emotional deprivation, an inability to influence their environment, and a fear of bodily harm. Studies of the former group of captives indicate that upon release they are often confused and suggestible; they have trouble concentrating or empathizing with the needs of others and experience bouts of severe anxiety and depression (Baker 1980). We regularly assume that prisoners of war or hostages will be substantially incapacitated when they return to freedom. No such assumption is made regarding jailed defendants in the course of criminal proceedings, even though they do not enjoy the advantage of having recently been freed, and they are haunted by the reality that their ordeal is just beginning.

Not all defendants, of course, are confined to jail before trial. Those who can afford bail may remain free and are likely to approach their trials with a more optimal level of anxiety than jailed defendants. Here opportunity and incapacity are interrelated. A lack of equal opportunity increases the psychological differences between defendants. Those who have the opportunity to stay out of jail are more likely to retain their psychological capacity to defend themselves.

3. Perfect defendants must be powerfully motivated to avoid punishment. They must be free of guilt for acts related or unre-

lated to the crime for which they are charged. They must also not be too concerned with the plight of codefendants. It is especially important that they have no need to ingratiate themselves with any of the participants in the trial procedure. Such needs might motivate them to acknowledge facts that are not in their favor. Perfect defendants must have an intense preoccupation with one and only one issue—their acquittal.

Psychiatrists and defense attorneys are often puzzled to find that some defendants are fatalistic regarding their defense and reluctant to do battle at trial even if they have a good defense. This behavior may be related to their guilt over what they have done or to the nature of the evidence against them, but it can also be partially understood as a manifestation of depression. Indeed, a considerable number of defendants experience symptoms of depression before they commit a crime (Halleck 1967). Most become depressed in the course of being arrested, indicted, and jailed. Depressed people tend to feel guilty. Sometimes they feel so guilty that they are willing to accept more punishment than society wants to impose. Or, they may accept a severe sentence simply because it allows them to be sent from jail to the relative safety of prison.

A sizable number of defendants who are not obviously depressed approach their trial with a sense of resignation and hopelessness. Poverty creates inequities here. Criminal defendants are often poor people who have learned to feel a sense of resignation in dealing with authority or the law. They rarely have the training, the inclination, or the emotional wherewithal to maximize their potential in the battle for exoneration.

4. Perfect defendants must project demeanors of innocence to the court. They must look sincere, honest, attractive, and likable. They must have the flexibility to project an aura of either confidence or despair. They must be likable but not ingratiating. They must project strength while convincing others that they have been victimized. All of this requires a sensitivity to the prevailing mood of others and considerable dramatic ability.

Defendants differ in their capacity to project an effective demeanor to the court. Many are severely handicapped. Those who are physically unattractive are at a distinct disadvantage. Conversely, especially attractive individuals may have an advantage. Other defendants simply lack the ability to project a favorable image. Anxiety also plays a role. Anxious defendants may appear "slippery" when they try too hard to prove their innocence, emotionally detached when they are simply paralyzed with fear, resentful when they are really ashamed and frightened, or aggressive when they are actually terrified. Other defendants simply lack the social or intellectual skills to make favorable impressions upon others.

Other inequities between defendants cannot be entirely understood by examining the psychology of individual defendants. One of the legal criteria for competency is the ability to consult with one's attorney with a reasonable degree of rational understanding. Two parties are involved in this process, and the efficiency of consultation will depend on the nature of their interaction. Attorneys, like defendants, vary in their personalities and capacities. A particular attorney may bring out the best in some clients and the worst in others. It usually matters whether attorneys like their clients, dislike them, or fear them. Defendants also respond differently to different attorneys. Those who distrust their attorneys, dislike them, or are sexually attracted to them may have diminished capacity to consult with them with a reasonable degree of rational understanding. Unconscious processes may also be at work in either party. If the attorney reminds the client of a previously disliked authority figure, it will be difficult for the client to consult effectively. The attorney who is repulsed by certain types of clients will have difficulty defending them.

Defendants will obviously be more competent if represented by some attorneys than by others. This is hardly a remarkable statement and by itself cannot be construed as questioning the fairness of the criminal justice process. Inequities do arise, however, from differences in opportunities to engage the most suitable attorney. Once again the wealthy are favored. They can hire the most experienced attorney, or they can shop around for a satisfactory "match." The indigent cannot choose their attorneys and must consult with those who may not be the most interested in their case or the most skilled. Sometimes a poor attorney-client match may in itself render the defendant functionally incompetent.

The above arguments elaborate a point made in the introductory chapter. Offenders differ markedly in their cognitive capacities, their levels of anxiety, their motivation to avoid punishment, and their ability to project an effective demeanor to the court. In the real world, perfect defendants rarely exist. A few may be very good, but most possess limited degrees of these qualities and skills. The incompetency decision, like all other adjudicatory devices that identify mentally disordered offenders, requires drawing a sharp line. A few defenders are declared incompetent and all others competent. Incompetent offenders can then be designated as exceptions that prove the rule. This pragmatic approach preserves the stability of a retributive system. It is sustained, however, only by ignoring realities of human psychology as they relate to the trial process.

While the arguments raised in this section may not justify major changes in society's approach to the incompetency issue, they still may have some practical implications for those who work in the criminal justice system. First, they should fuel continued interest in improving conditions in our jails. To the extent that defendants are severely traumatized in jail and do not have ready access to the services of mental health professionals, they will have impaired competency to proceed in the criminal justice system and will be at risk of receiving more punishment than they "deserve." Second, the foregoing arguments should alert defense attorneys to the psychological needs of their clients during criminal proceedings. Attorneys can do a better job of defending their clients if they are aware of their clients' cognitive and emotional impairments. Such awareness may influence decisions to seek delays, to refer clients for mental health treatment, to accept clients' consent to a negotiated plea, or to put clients on the witness stand. Defense attorneys in the criminal justice process must be counselors as well as advocates. To the extent that they are aware of their clients' handicaps, they will be more effective in this role.

How Does the Incompetency Diversion Affect Public Safety?

While the incompetency diversion appears to have been developed as a beneficent device for protecting defendants, society is also concerned with its use for the public safety. In the pre-*Jackson* era, supposedly dangerous individuals were restrained under the incompetency diversion for long periods to protect the public. Whatever protection was thereby provided is less available in the modern era, but no substantial diminution of public protection has occurred since the *Jackson* decision. Incompetent defendants who are felt to be dangerous and mentally ill can, as a rule, be civilly committed. (Even though these individuals may not have been proven to have committed a dangerous act in criminal court, they may still meet the criteria for civil commitment.) Problems are most likely to arise in those rare instances where defendants cannot be committed because their incompetence is not related to mental illness (e.g., deafness or mutism). Even this contingency has been overcome in some states through statutes with special provisions for civil commitment of unrestorable incompetents who are believed to be dangerous (Parker 1975). Some reassurance that the incompetency plea has little negative influence on public safety can also be found in surveys that show the recidivism rates of pretrial incompetents, once released, to be very similar to those of released prisoners (Mowbray 1979; Steadman 1979). These studies also reveal that only a small number of incompetent defendants were subsequently arrested for crimes against persons.

The quest for increased public protection is often linked to efforts to rehabilitate offenders. It might be assumed that incompetent defendants treated with the variety of techniques available to mental health professionals would, upon release, make a better social adjustment. Unfortunately, while the recidivism rate of these persons is no higher than that of prisoners convicted of the same crime and later released, it is still quite high. Furthermore, as many as 50 percent of the incompetent group may be rehospitalized at a later time (Mowbray 1979). Thus, while the treatments used with incompetents may succeed in achieving the primary objective of returning them to court, they appear to have little long-term influence on their deviant behavior. There is no evidence at this point that rehabilitative efforts with incompetent defendants have a positive influence on public safety.

Clinical Issues

Assessment of Competency by Mental Health Professionals

Do mental health professionals who evaluate offenders have sufficient skills to relate their knowledge of human behavior and mental illness to the legal criteria by which mentally disordered offenders are identified? Most mental health professionals and attorneys, as well as most of the public, would say yes. At the same time, a substantial scholarly literature questions whether psychiatric and psychological concepts of diagnosis and treatment of mental illness are actually relevant to the determination of competency (Jeffery 1967; Szasz 1963). In view of the difference between popular belief and academic skepticism, it is useful to review what mental health professionals actually learn about competency in the course of their training and practice.

Competency can be defined as the ability or capacity to do a task. Sometimes the task involves conduct, such as driving an automobile. Sometimes it involves making a choice. In ordinary clinical settings, mental health professionals evaluate their patients' competency daily. They decide whether patients should attend therapeutic functions, leave the ward, or assume a variety of obligations on the ward, such as keeping track of appointments or medications. The issues here are whether patients have the capacity to perform such tasks with sufficient skill so as not to diminish their already compromised self-esteem by failing, or whether they can perform them without harming themselves or disrupting the ward. If patients lack these capacities, they are judged incompetent to perform such tasks. In the outpatient setting, similar judgments are ordinarily made concerning the extent to which patients can be allowed to assume certain responsibilities, like monitoring their own medications.

These days, the interest of clinicians in determining competency has been enhanced by litigation dealing with the patient's right to refuse treatment. With few exceptions, patients can be treated against their will only when they are found to be incompetent. This rule has always existed, but only in recent years has it been strictly enforced. Mental health clinicians are called upon with increasing frequency to evaluate the competency of patients to make decisions regarding treatment (*Rogers v. Okin* 1980).

Mental health professionals are also regularly bombarded with requests from various agencies for opinions as to whether individuals who have received psychological treatment or who are currently in treatment can perform certain tasks such as holding down a job, driving a car, or attending school. The wisdom of clinicians making such assessments is debatable, but the large number of requests for evaluation suggests that many administrators trust such evaluations. And certainly many mental health professionals assume the task of evaluating a wide variety of capacities. Generally, clinicians are best at assessing competency to perform tasks with which they are familiar. It is relatively easy, for example, to predict that depressed patients will not be competent participants in group activities that require a great deal of communication, concentration, and energy. On the other hand, it is much harder for clinicians to determine how patients, even those with serious illnesses, will perform as drivers, military officers, or government employees.

The common-sense observation that evaluations of competency to perform a task are more accurate when examiners are familiar with the task may have some important ramifications for pretrial incompetency diversion in the criminal justice system. Attorneys are likely to have special skills in determining whether defendants have "sufficient present ability to consult with their defense attorney with a reasonable degree of rational understanding." They, in fact, may be more skilled at such assessments than mental health clinicians. Attorneys should know how much communication with a client is necessary to prepare a satisfactory defense. They know what type of information they need to prepare an effective case and can probably judge accurately whether the client can provide it. They also have a good idea of what type of defense is likely to have the greatest chance of success. Having attorneys assist mental health clinicians in assessing capacities would lend much more precision to the evaluation process.

Ultimately, an assessment of competency is a prediction that an individual will be able to perform a given task, at a certain time, under certain circumstances. Such predictions are inevitably biased by the clinician's training, experience, and values. One obvious bias is in the direction of assuming the competency of those who are pleasant and cooperative. Clinicians usually assume that those who consent to their requests have made rational choices and that those who refuse have not. In effect, they judge the client's rationality by comparing it with their own. (Such bias is not peculiar to mental health professionals. Attorneys are also unlikely to raise the issue of incompetency as long as their clients are cooperative.)

Some realistic aspects of the predicting situation move the biases of clinicians toward conservatism. Feedback as to the accuracy of clinical predictions of incompetency is rarely available. Once individuals are judged incompetent to perform a certain task, they are usually prevented from doing it. There is therefore no way of knowing if the initial judgment was correct. Controlled studies in which people are given the opportunity to perform a task they have been judged incompetent to perform have not been done. The only occasions when clinicians obtain data that question their biases are when individuals "slip through the system" and successfully complete tasks which they would have been prohibited from attempting. On the other hand, predictions of competency might also provide clinicians with discouraging feedback. When clients fail a task they have been judged to be able to master, clinicians learn to demand a higher level of capacity in predicting the competency of future clients.

The assessment of competency may be a poorly conceptualized and inadequately studied skill, but it is nevertheless a function mental health professionals must perform in everyday clinical practice. It should not be too much, therefore, to ask them to describe how various intellectual and emotional dysfunctions might compromise the capacity of defendants to consult with a lawyer and have a reasonable degree of understanding of courtroom proceedings. The legal issues may be somewhat remote from the everyday experience of clinical practice, but the basic process of assessment of capacity is not.

Restoration of Competency

The major task facing those who care for incompetent offenders is relatively straightforward: to restore the competency of defendants as quickly as possible. Given current tendencies to view quite handicapped persons as competent, it is not too difficult to help most defendants achieve sufficient improvement so that they can return to the criminal justice process.

Two factors inherent in the diversion process favor the restoration of competency. First, the time involved in the evaluation may be sufficient to allow the disorders of some defendants to spontaneously remit. The likelihood of this happening is increased when defendants are housed in safe environments where they are treated, at least some of the time, as individuals in need of help rather than punishment. Second, most serious mental disorders, with the exception of some organic brain disorders and mental retardation, are either reversible or remitting. The odds favor defendants with schizophrenic or affective disorders, who will often improve as long as they are treated humanely.

Modern treatment of mental disorders, especially treatment with drugs, is highly effective in the short run. Symptoms can be controlled to a sufficient degree to allow defendants to manage their lives in a rational manner. When pharmacological therapy is accompanied by psychotherapy, the chances of recovery are even greater. Some institutions have also developed special programs for incompetent defendants that teach them about criminal trial procedures and give them an opportunity to rehearse the role of defendant. Such direct efforts to expand the capacities of defendants to deal with the issues of adjudication can be very useful.

Some jurists question whether defendants restored to capacity by psychotropic medication should be returned to court as competent. Many of these individuals would probably lose their new-found competency if they stopped taking medication. They might also project an unfavorable image if their medication caused them to look too disturbed or tranquil. Such considerations have led some courts to question the "synthetic sanity" of those restored to competency by medicine (*State v. Hayes* 1978). These concerns are unrealistic. Remissions of mental illness or other behavioral change resulting from pharmacotherapy are no more synthetic than remissions of physical illness treated with drugs such as digitalis or insulin. The likelihood that psychotropic drugs will markedly alter the defendant's appearance is usually greatly exaggerated by those not familiar with the effects of these agents. The major problem in using pharmacotherapy, particularly with psychotic defendants, is ensuring that they receive and take their medicine. Medication may not be readily available when they return to the jail setting. Side effects of some medications may also be distressing to defendants and thus discourage their use, while termination of pharmacotherapy will frequently bring about a return of the psychosis.

Emerging Legal Issues

Legal conflicts concerning the incompetency diversion usually involve disputes as to whether such practices enhance public protection or protect the rights of defendants. As in most areas of law, these conflicts reflect changes in the prevailing moral and political climate of the community. In the early 1970s, the mental health field was in large part dominated by a libertarian movement. Most of the litigation regarding mentally disordered offenders at that time was directed to preserving their rights. In the 1980s, when fear of crime has become a major societal concern, the emphasis has shifted to providing the public with greater protection, with a consequent shift in legislation toward more restriction on mentally disordered offenders.

Any understanding of current controversies is complicated by differences in the procedures that determine the disposition of mentally disordered offenders from one state to another. Federal circuit court decisions may lead to changes in only one jurisdiction. Even Supreme Court decisions are implemented slowly, and the statutes they spawn are characterized by many variations designed to meet local needs. This makes it difficult to determine how a widespread or general legal controversy is influencing defendants in any particular jurisdiction.

This section provides a brief review of some of the legal issues regarding incompetent defendants that are currently receiving a considerable degree of attention. I will make no effort to predict how current controversies will be resolved. The future legal controversies involving mentally disordered offenders will be determined by economic and political changes as well as by the development of new technologies for treatment. In this area, too many variables are involved for anyone to be sanguine about their conjectural skills.

One interesting trend comes from a shift in court administrative policy that expands the liberty of incompetent defendants. The courts are increasingly willing to allow competency examinations to be made in the community rather than in distant hospitals, to insist that examinations be completed as quickly as possible, and to allow the defendant the right to bail while competency is being determined. There is also a trend toward allowing defendants already adjudicated incompetent to be treated on a outpatient basis. Some of this change is supported by emergence of the "less restrictive alternative" doctrine, which mandates that the needs of public safety be served with the minimum sacrifice of clients' rights (Singer 1972). Such change may also have a more practical motivation. The courts have come to appreciate that community evaluation and treatment of those accused of nonviolent crimes can often be done safely, expeditiously, and cost-effectively. Saving money without jeopardizing the public serves as an important reinforcer of less restrictive dispositions.

It is unclear whether any trend is emerging regarding the rights of incompetent defendants to receive or to refuse treatment. Litigation of the right to treatment has moved along ponderously in both public mental hospitals and security hospitals, although in some instances it has resulted in substantial improvement of facilities (Stone 1977). Incompetent defendants may have an especially strong case for a right to treatment since the *Jackson* decision makes their continued restraint contingent on progress in treatment (*Jackson v. Indiana* 1972). The right to refuse treatment, which has created so much concern among those who work in public mental hospitals, does not appear to be as powerful a problem in security hospitals that treat incompetent defendants. The state has a substantial interest in bringing incompetent defendants to trial as quickly as possible. This interest might outweigh whatever interest defendants may have in refusing treatment that would restore their competency (Wilnick 1977).

Expanded legal interest can be hoped for but probably not expected in two other areas. One involves the issue of defendants' incompetency at the time of plea negotiation. I have noted earlier that a large number of defendants are especially vulnerable to mental disorder at the time of plea negotiation and may make irrational decisions in accepting pleas. Defense attorneys can do something about this problem, either by asking for more determinations of competency at the time of plea negotiation or by becoming more aware of their clients' handicaps and providing them with more intensive treatment or counseling.

More dialogue is also needed in relating the nature of expert testimony to standards of incompetency. All the adjudications that identify mentally disordered offenders are based on legal standards of competency, sanity, dangerousness, or mental illness. These standards are not couched in the language of mental health professionals but in language that can be understood by jurors. The standards are always broad and never specify what degree of incapacity is required to initiate diversion. The *Dusky* standard, for example, deals with whether the defendant has "sufficient present ability to consult with his attorney with a reasonable degree of rational understanding." The term "sufficient" is not defined. Judges or jurors are given considerable latitude in deciding which moral or social as well as psychological issues to use in deciding when defendants are "sufficiently" impaired. When experts testify in a conclusory manner as to what is "sufficient," it can be argued that they are presenting a moral rather than a medical or psychological opinion and are, therefore, usurping the function of the judge or jury.

Most of the criticism of the practice of experts in providing conclusory testimony has been directed toward insanity cases or predictions of dangerousness (Shah 1974; Monahan 1981). Here, experts have been urged to provide the court with whatever information is available and in as much detail as possible, without responding to the legal standard to which the adjudication is addressed. The hope is that judges or juries, once fully cognizant of the expert's information, will make a final decision based primarily on the moral wishes or the conscience of the community. Experts can easily provide nonconclusory testimony in pretrial incompetency cases. A number of checklists are available that allow experts to make appropriate evaluations of various incapacities relative to the defendant's ability to proceed (McGarry et al. 1973). Experts could simply report these evaluations to the court without drawing conclusions.

The most intense legal controversies involving the incompetency diversion are around the issue of abolishing or modifying the process. Morris (1982), the most noteworthy proponent of abolishing certain aspects of the incompetency diversion, now proposes that the defendant's capacity be approached in the following manner:

The plea of incompetency to stand trial should be changed. A motion of trial continuance by reason of disability should be allowed up to a maximum of 6 months for the accused to maximize his fitness for trial. Psychiatric and psychological (or other) treatment, where appropriate, should be made available to him to this end during this period in the least restrictive setting determined by the court. Thereafter, at the election of the prosecution, either the trial should proceed on the rules of court designed so far as practicable to re-dress the trial disadvantages under which the accused labors or a *nolle prosequi* should be entered. In making this selection there would be no impropriety in the state's first pursuing civil commitment processes against the accused, it being understood that the prosecution will proceed to trial only if the accused is not civilly committed.

Morris' proposal would allow for a trial of the unrestorable incompetent who is potentially dangerous. Special rules would be invoked to compensate for the handicaps of defendants. These would give defendants certain advantages in the process of discovery. The jury would be instructed to make no inference from the courtroom demeanor of defendants or their failure to testify. Provisions to expedite a new trial would be available if new evidence should be discovered. Morris' proposal might not meet constitutional requirements, but if it did, more defendants could be brought to court quickly and the possibility of prolonged institutionalization of incompetent defendants in public mental hospitals or security hospitals would be eliminated.

Other proposals for modifying the incompetency diversion stop short of abolition. A few states have developed procedures that allow for "acquittal only" or "innocent only" trials in which defendants who might have been found incompetent are allowed to face their charges in court. If acquitted they are freed; if convicted and later found incompetent, the verdict is set aside (Roesch and Golding 1979).

CHAPTER 4

Offenders Found Not Guilty
by Reason of Insanity

OUR LEGAL SYSTEM ASSUMES that most individuals who violate the criminal law have a rational capacity for choice and therefore possess free will. Because they have chosen to do wrong, they are assumed to be responsible for their actions and are appropriate subjects for punishment. For centuries, however, Anglo-American law has also provided a means for excusing from punishment offenders who lack understanding of their actions or who appear unable to control them. Those who commit crimes as a result of a legally recognized "mistake" or "duress" may be excused, as also are infants (i.e., children below the age of 7 years). Anglo-American law also acknowledges that certain mental disorders so impair understanding and the capacity to make choices that those afflicted cannot be held responsible for their criminal conduct. Their exculpation is accomplished through the insanity defense, which, if successful, relieves them of all responsibility for the crime. These "acquittees" may then be subjected to indeterminate periods of hospitalization.

Identification and Disposition of Defendants
Found Not Guilty by Reason of Insanity

Purpose of the Insanity Defense

Perhaps the most succinct summary of the purpose of the insanity defense appears in a statement by Judge David Bazelon in his opinion in *Durham v. United States* (1954). Bazelon stated that "our collective conscience does not allow punishment where it cannot impose blame."

The insanity defense is sometimes viewed as modifying the mental element or *mens rea* (guilty mind) that must be present at the time of the criminal act if the perpetrator is to be found guilty. In this view, the presence of a serious mental illness at the time of the crime may preclude the requisite legal intent to commit that crime. The insanity defense, however, is not always related to the question of intent. It may also be viewed as an affirmative defense in which criminal intent is acknowledged but where criminal sanctions may not be justly imposed because the defendant claims a mental disorder impaired his capacity to choose. This distinction has important procedural consequences in law. When insanity is viewed as a matter of *mens rea* or criminal intent, the burden of persuasion is generally on the state to prove the defendant's sanity beyond a reasonable doubt. When the insanity defense is viewed as an affirmative defense, the burden is generally upon defendants to prove their insanity by a preponderance of or clear and convincing evidence (depending on the particular jurisdiction).

Most legal scholars believe that the insanity defense strengthens the criminal justice system by restricting exculpation to only the most severely impaired, thereby implying that all other defendants are to be held responsible for their actions (Stone 1975). Without the insanity defense and the assumption that all sane defendants are responsible for their acts, psychological issues might have to be considered in the assessment of every offender's liability. This would not only burden the criminal justice system but might also diminish whatever benefits society gains when it labels lawbreakers as blameworthy.

Who Raises the Insanity Defense and Who Is Found Insane?

The number of defendants who successfully plead the insanity defense and thus are defined as mentally disordered offenders is relatively small. Only a fraction of 1 percent of felony cases results in acquittal by reason of insanity (Pasewark 1981). The insanity defense tends to be disproportionately raised by defendants charged with crimes that carry severe penalties, such as criminal homicide. Demographically, those found not guilty by reason of insanity are somewhat different from other offenders. They tend to be older and are more likely to be Caucasian and of middle-class social status. Society is also inclined to excuse those who do not fit its usual stereotype of criminals, such as police officers who commit violent crimes or mothers who attempt to murder their children (Pasewark 1981).

An acquittal by reason of insanity does not ordinarily allow defendants to go free, even though they have, in theory, committed no crime. Other legal mechanisms unrelated to the issue of culpability are invoked in an effort to restrain them. Traditionally, society has feared that those acquitted may be dangerous; hence, it has created laws that allow for their continued confinement and treatment, usually in maximum security hospitals. While in recent years insanity acquittees have had greater opportunities to be set free or sent to a civil hospital, most still spend several months to years in institutions housing other mentally disordered offenders.

In 1978, insanity acquittees accounted for approximately 8 percent of admissions to these facilities. Because they tend to stay for longer periods than other mentally disordered offenders (particularly those found incompetent to stand trial), they account for a larger percentage of the institutionalized mentally disordered offender population. In 1978, they made up 22 percent of that population (Steadman and Braff 1983). In terms of numbers, insanity acquittees do not have the same impact on the criminal justice system as those found incompetent to stand trial. From the standpoint of institutions that must care for them, however, this group may create sizable problems.

Some understanding of why insanity acquittees make up an unusually troubling group may be gleaned by considering the exact nature of the insanity defense. This defense deals only with the mental states of defendants at the time of their crimes. Their mental status before or after the crime, including their mental status at the time of trial, is not relevant to the assessment of blameworthiness. In order to be tried, defendants must have sufficient mental capacity to be found competent to stand trial. Achievement of this status would tend to preclude the possibility that such defendants are gravely disturbed at the time they are tried and acquitted. Thus, institutions dealing with insanity acquittees generally confront individuals whose mental disturbances are in remission. This contrasts with the mental status of those confined because of incompetency to stand trial, who are likely to be more acutely impaired. By the time insanity acquittees reach the hospital, they may show few signs of mental illness and may not be motivated to seek treatment. With the exception of mentally disordered sex offenders, they are likely to be the most psychologically intact patients within the institution. Since many of them have antisocial tendencies, they may resist the authority of the staff or become predatory to other inmates.

Standards for Determining Insanity

Depending on the jurisdiction, two major standards or tests determine insanity in the United States—the *M'Naghten* test and the American Law Institute (ALI) test. These tests are designed to guide the jury in assessing when the defendant's mental illness and the resulting impairment are severe enough to preclude the ascription of criminal blame or culpability.

According to the *M'Naghten* test,

> Every man is presumed to be sane, and . . . to establish a defense on the ground of insanity it must be clearly proved that at the time of the committing of the act, the party accused was laboring under such a defect of reason from disease of the mind, as not to know the nature and quality of the act he was doing or if he did know it, that he did not know he was doing what was wrong. (*M'Naghten's Case* 1843)

The quest for an excuse here can be paraphrased as "I did not know what I was doing" or "I did not know what I did was wrong."

According to the American Law Institute test,

> A person is not responsible for criminal conduct if at the time of such conduct as a result of mental disease or defect he lacked substantial capacity either to appreciate the criminality of his conduct or to conform his conduct to the requirements of the law. (American Law Institute 1962)

This test includes elements of "I didn't know what I was doing or that it was wrong," but adds the volitional element, "I couldn't control my behavior." The ALI test also differs from the *M'Naghten* test in using two terms susceptible to broad interpretation, namely, "substantial" and "appreciate." It does not demand a finding of total lack of knowledge or appreciation for exculpation but only a "substantial" lack of capacity. By using the term "appreciate" rather than "know," it also allows for consideration of emotional incapacities that may influence understanding.

Whether the use of the "liberal" ALI test allows for the presentation of more information to the jury or results in more acquittals is unknown. The available data suggest that the nature of the standards does not significantly alter psychiatric testimony and appears to have little influence on trial outcome (Pasewark 1981). It would seem logical that the nature of the standard would ultimately influence the number of acquittees, however, and some evidence supports this view. During the 1950s, when the very "liberal" *Durham* rule was the standard in the District of Columbia, a noticeable increase in acquittals occurred (Rennie 1978). [The *Durham* rule stated that "an accused is not criminally responsible if his unlawful criminal conduct was the product of a mental disease or mental defect" (*Durham v. United States* 1954). This standard was found objectionable by jurors and legislators and after a few years was replaced by the ALI test (Brooks 1974).]

Until the trial of the attempted Presidential assassin John Hinckley, Jr., many jurisdictions liberalized insanity standards and replaced *M'Naghten* with the ALI standard. The acquittal of Hinckley seems to have catalyzed a trend in the opposite direction. Three states (Montana in 1979, Idaho in 1982, and Utah in 1983) abolished the insanity defense, and some others have made efforts to do so. Some states that currently use the ALI standard are considering a return to the *M'Naghten* standard, believing that its use will result in fewer acquittals. Even the American Psychiatric Association, which once lobbied for more liberal standards, recently endorsed the following standard, which is very close to *M'Naghten*.

A person charged with a criminal offense should be found not guilty by reason of insanity if it is shown that as a result of mental disease or mental retardation he was unable to appreciate the wrongfulness of his conduct at the time of the offense. (Bonnie 1982)

The Insanity Defense Reform Act of 1984 (part of the Comprehensive Crime Control Act of 1984) brought about some major changes in the federal criminal code and has significantly modified and tightened the standards for exculpatory insanity in federal courts. The new federal insanity test states:

It is an affirmative defense to a prosecution under any federal statute that, at the time of the commission of the acts constituting the offense, the defendant, as a result of severe mental disease or defect, was unable to appreciate the nature and quality or the wrongfulness of his acts.

The new federal law also requires defendants who wish to raise the defense of insanity to assume the burden of proving this defense by a standard of clear and convincing evidence. Moreover, by amending the Federal Rules of Evidence, the nature and scope of expert testimony on the ultimate legal issues have also been restricted.

Society's concern with finding the "best" standard for determining insanity can be viewed as a reflection of its uncertainty regarding the extent to which it wishes to allow mental illness to be an exculpatory factor. With the exception of a few years' experimentation with the *Durham* rule, society has consistently sought a standard that is sufficiently narrow as to excuse only a small number of offenders who have serious mental illnesses.

Role and Problems of Mental Health Professionals

In the process of determining insanity, the criminal justice system almost always requests the assistance of psychiatrists and psychologists. They are asked to evaluate defendants some time after the crime has taken place and to speculate about their mental condition at the time of the crime. If the examiners believe the defendant was mentally ill at the time of the crime, they must also try to speculate if that degree of illness was sufficient to justify exculpation under the *M'Naghten*, ALI, or other standards. These are extremely difficult tasks. Even if defendants appear to be mentally ill at the time of the insanity examination, it is not easy to determine if this illness was present or if it in fact exerted significant influence upon them at the time of their crimes. If clinicians believe that the illness of defendants played a role in compromising their capacity for free choice, they must also make what is essentially a moral judgment as to the degree of disability that exculpates or negates blameworthiness. Much disagreement is likely among mental health professionals in making such a judgment. They may, as professionals, agree on the degree of the defendant's disability; as individuals who hold different moral standards, however, they may well disagree about whether that degree of disability should exculpate (Goldstein 1967).

The insanity trial is often characterized as a "battle of experts" (Slovenko 1973). This depiction is rarely accurate. In occasional and usually well-publicized cases, mental health experts employed by the defense and the prosecution will disagree about whether the degree of the defendant's disability is sufficient to preclude criminal responsibility. On even rarer occasions, they may disagree about the extent or the nature of the defendant's disability at the time of the offense. The majority of insanity trials, however, do not feature disagreement among mental health experts. Often the issue of insanity is not even contested by the prosecution. Only one expert, usually a court-appointed and allegedly neutral clinician, may examine the patient. (Usually that expert is a state employee who is also charged with assessing the defendant's competency to stand trial.) Prosecution and defense attorneys, particularly when dealing with indigent clients, rarely seek the services of adversarial expert witnesses to contest the findings of state-employed experts. As a rule, the court hears only one expert opinion and will rely on it heavily in making its determination.

Postacquittal Disposition

Society's concerns with the insanity defense have recently been complicated by legal changes influencing the disposition of acquittees. Up until the early 1970s, the disposition of insanity acquittees was relatively straightforward and, from the standpoint of the public, noncontroversial. A very few individuals, usually respected citizens or females (or both), were actually released upon acquittal. The overwhelming majority were sent to institutions for mentally disordered offenders, where they tended to remain for long periods of time. Often, acquittees were confined for a period of time roughly comparable with, or even exceeding, that which they would have served if convicted. In cases involving homicide, where defendants might have received a lifetime sentence if convicted, they tended to be confined in maximum security hospitals for at least 10 years.

In the 1970s, some jurisdictions began to alter this practice significantly and to provide insanity acquittees with the same legal protection and the same opportunities for release as those committed under civil statutes. In the past several years, such changes have created a great deal of societal concern and have resulted in litigation and legislation to restore some of the restraints that used to be applied to insanity acquittees. Concern with the possible release of insane offenders has also resulted in a new plea of "guilty but mentally ill." Some of the recent problems in determining the disposition of insanity acquittees, which have complex legal origins, will be discussed in greater detail in a subsequent section.

Legal Issues

Social and Legal Functions of Blaming and Excusing

Responsibility is a hypothetical quality society attributes to individuals in determining the morality of their conduct. Society's fundamental objective in imposing blame and punishment is the regulation of social behavior. When we believe people have the capacity to choose, we evaluate their conduct as blameworthy or praiseworthy. When we blame people for doing things we do not like, we usually impose punishment. In many social situations, this consequence may simply be verbal condemnation or withdrawal of reinforcement. In criminal law, the consequence, in addition to the stigma of a conviction, is likely to be a powerful punishment involving loss of freedom or, less frequently, loss of wealth.

The insanity defense is perhaps the most thoroughly studied social process pertaining to the issue of responsibility. (I am using "responsibility" here to imply moral accountability or blameworthiness for past conduct. The term is frequently used with related but slightly different meanings. Sometimes it refers to a moral obligation for future conduct, e.g., "you are responsible for taking care of your brother." This admonition implies that conduct that fails to meet obligations is blameworthy. Sometimes responsibility implies causality, e.g., "this bad weather is making me crabby." Here, blameworthiness is attributed to a cause outside of the individual.)

The issue of responsibility covers more, of course, than simply deciding whether criminals should be blamed or excused. The question of whether we should blame, praise, or excuse people for their actions arises in all aspects of human life. In raising and educating children, in doing psychotherapy, or in governing society, someone must decide when individuals will be blamed or excused. In making these decisions, those who judge must consider many characteristics of those who are to be judged, including their physical and mental disabilities. Viewed in this light, the insanity defense is not an isolated or unfamiliar issue. It is, rather, the most dramatic example society can provide of how society considers the existence of certain disabilities in assessing blameworthiness.

Not all antisocial acts are blameworthy or deserving of punishment. The criminal justice system must, therefore, define the conditions under which offenders may be excused from punishment and provide some guidelines about how this must be done. In our system of justice, illegal conduct does not in itself constitute a crime. To be found guilty of a crime, an offender must have an evil or guilty state of mind (*mens rea*). Conviction for most crimes is impossible without this mental element and voluntary illegal conduct (*actus reus*) (Perkins 1969). Guided by this doctrine, our criminal justice system will not always invoke punishment against those who have committed a crime in various legally recognized and defined circumstances, such as self-defense, under duress, or by accident. And, as already noted, it will also, at times, excuse the insane—those who at the time of the crime lacked the requisite comprehension of their actions or the requisite ability to control them.

In the modern era, our courts have rarely been concerned with the mental state of an offender as an exculpatory factor unless that state can be characterized as a disability sufficiently severe as to meet the legal standards defining insanity. The *mens rea* or mental element accompanying a crime has become narrowly defined, so that simple awareness of conduct, the circumstances under which it occurs, and its probable consequences are usually sufficient to assume intent or a guilty mind (Kadish and Paulsen 1975). Past experiences, motivations for committing the crime, social circumstances, physical health, and other psychological variables are largely irrelevant for the purpose of determining guilt. Nor is the determination of guilt influenced by evidence that the behavior of the defendant in the course of the crime was of such a nature that most people would have judged it irrational. These factors may be taken into consideration in the sentencing process, but they do not negate guilt or criminal liability (Hermann 1983).

In restricting consideration of mental disability to the insanity defense when determining guilt or liability, the criminal justice system treats the issue of the responsibility of the mentally disordered in an "all or none" manner. A few are excused, and all others are considered fully responsible. The statutorily prescribed punishment associated with the ascription of responsibility is graded according to the seriousness of the offense, not the characteristics of the actor. It is noteworthy that this approach differs significantly from the manner in which responsibility is assessed in other social situations.

In most social situations, we tend to evaluate the issue of responsibility according to personal characteristics of individuals. We think in terms of degrees or gradations of responsibility and will consider a large number of variables in mitigating punishment. In deciding how to punish children, for example, parents and teachers consider the motivation of children and the influence of whatever physical and emotional stresses they might be experiencing. In demanding that patients take responsibility for inappropriate or antisocial behavior, therapists modify the nature and extent of demands they place on patients according to their perception of the degree of their mental and physical impairments. When people fail to meet obligations, such as paying their bills or coming to work on time, creditors and employers may consider a variety of social and biological incapacities as setting limits on the ease with which they will impose sanctions against them.

Historical Bases for Limiting Excuses Based on Mental Disability

The particular manner in which the criminal justice system relates impairment to the ascription of blame is best understood from a historical perspective. Our legal system was not developed with the intention of relating punishment to the criminal, but rather to the crime. Prior to the 19th century, little attention was paid to the causes of crime, and consequently little need existed to look at the differences in the social background, the biology, or the psychology of offenders that may have played a role in their crimes (Rennie 1978).

The primary problem for society has always been to determine what to do about crime, and this problem was largely confronted without considering the causes of crime. If asked the reasons why people commit crime, most legal theorists of the 18th century, and perhaps many now, would probably say that they do it out of greed, weakness, or evil. All these "explanations" assume free choice and justify a judgment of blameworthiness. Under this view of criminal behavior, responsibility is assessed primarily on the basis of the defendant's behavior, and all offenders who have done the same act under the same circumstances are equally guilty. A "just deserts" response to crime then appears rational, and punishment can be simply related to the degree of harm the offender has inflicted on society.

In the latter part of the 18th century, the process of justice began to be dominated by more utilitarian goals. This was the "Age of Reason," in which liberal scholars such as Jeremy Bentham developed a view of punishment that was based largely on the prin-

ciple of deterrence (Bentham 1948). According to the historian
Rennie (1978):

> To eighteenth century thinkers, the criminal was a rational
> being who could precisely calculate his chances of detection
> and quantum of punishment and decide, "This crime is worth
> committing; that crime is not." If this were, indeed, the fact,
> then the calculus of hedonism could be as precisely plotted as
> the trajectory of the planets, making possible, for the first
> time, a rational system of criminal justice. (p. 22)

In this school of jurisprudence, more emphasis was placed on
certainty than on severity of punishment. The classical criminolo-
gist believed it was necessary to impose a penalty only severe
enough to outweigh the probable benefits the defendant might
perceive in the criminal act. Any penalty in excess of this amount
was considered wasteful.

Rennie also notes that the following principles derived from
18th century liberalism have continued to exert critical influence
in European and American criminal law:

> That man is a rational being; that he avoids pain and pursues
> pleasure; that the criminal law should impose such sanctions
> that will outweigh the rewards of crime; that sanctions should
> be announced in advance; that they should be proportional to
> the offense; that everyone should enjoy equal justice; and that
> what a man does, not what he thinks, is the proper ambit of
> the criminal law. (p. 24)

As with the "just deserts" principle, the deterrence principle
provides a guide for dealing with crime based on assumptions that
rational motivations, such as greed or lust, explain crime. All offenders who commit the same crime under the same circumstances
are equally responsible and can, in theory, be deterred by the
same degree of punishment.

At the time, supporters advocated that important advantages
were associated with the desert/deterrence model, sometimes
referred to as the classical school of criminology. Dealing with the
crime rather than the criminal increased the likelihood of a fair
approach to retribution in a society that was often characterized
by unequal treatment before the law. Justice in the 18th century

was not the same for the nobleman, the tradesman, and the peasant. The classical approach to criminology was in large part associated with a movement to break down the oppression of class rule and to provide equal justice in society. To an arguable extent, it succeeded in that goal, and it is still viewed as the most equitable approach to the problem of criminal behavior.

The theoretical underpinnings of the desert-deterrence model began to be questioned during the latter part of the 18th century. With the development of statistical methods, criminologists became aware that crime was not distributed throughout society in a random manner (which would be expected if its main determinants were simply greed or lust). Instead, it was found that offenders could be characterized by a prevalence of certain qualities that distinguished them from nonoffenders. They were more likely to come from certain localities and to have certain socioeconomic characteristics. In the 19th and 20th centuries, many more social differences between offenders and others were noted. Meanwhile, behavioral scientists also began to describe a large variety of biological and psychological variations among those who had committed crimes (Rennie 1978).

All of these new data made it possible to derive explanations of crime based on causal factors that could not be conceptualized as always under the control of the offender. It is difficult to know how much blameworthiness a society should impose upon offenders who, through no fault of their own, have serious biological or social handicaps that may be causally related to their crimes. Social and biological explanations of crime force society to reconsider the assumptions that all offenders are rational and blameworthy. They also force society to acknowledge that major biological and social differences may exist between offenders who commit the same act, and that these differences may reflect degrees of handicaps that might warrant attributing to these offenders gradations of blameworthiness and also of punishment.

While at times during the past century biological, sociological, and psychological determinism have had a considerable influence on the criminal justice system, they have never made an appreciable dent in its method of assessing liability. Society continues to stress the crime rather than the criminal. New theories of crime and new data as to the nature of criminals have sometimes influenced the process of sentencing or the manner in which convicted offenders are treated. But even at those times when a substantial number of criminologists have believed that a particular social, biological, or psychological factor was a major cause of crimes, the influence of that factor at the time of the crime has been given little consideration in the assessment of liability.

Considering Individual Differences in Imposing Punishment

Certain practical reasons are given for excluding scientific knowledge of individual differences from the guilt assessment phase of criminal justice. Those who defend the current system make the following arguments:

1. Explanations of criminality can in themselves be viewed as exculpatory. Conduct that seems to be understood is often excused. If too much is excused, then not enough is deemed blameworthy, and the assumption of choice or free will is challenged. Should the number of offenders found incapable of choosing become a substantial minority or majority of the law-breaking population, a system of justice that relies heavily on retribution would no longer make sense.
2. Current scientific explanations of crime can all be challenged. No theory of crime has been proven. The available factual data about crime are probably insufficient to assist the courts in assessing blame.
3. Consideration of scientific variables in assessing liability of every offender could lead to a system of ascribing guilt that would require the court to assess the degree of disability in every case. This would be an extremely expensive and time-consuming task.
4. The law would lose its fairness if it relied on individualized judgments of culpability and punishment. Under such a system, it would be difficult to develop general standards of judgment, and too many arbitrary decisions might allow guilty offenders to avoid punishment altogether.
5. If liability were viewed in terms of individual variation, it is likely that more offenders would receive shorter sentences or perhaps no sentences. Some of those excused might be the most dangerous. This would jeopardize public safety.

Some of these arguments are powerful and, for the most part, they have been persuasive in keeping considerations of psychological and other sciences out of the guilt assessment process. A constant tension exists, however, between the criminal justice system's assumption of the sameness of all individuals who commit similar acts in similar circumstances and society's awareness of marked sociological, psychological, and biological differences among defendants. Periodically, new legal doctrines allow an increased amount of data relating to the science of human behavior to seep into the criminal justice system and influence its assessment of culpability. Sometimes this is accomplished by broadening the scope of the insanity defense. The legal system may make it easier, for example, for a defendant to gain an acquittal by changing the standards that determine insanity. This may involve demanding only "substantial" rather than full capacity to know or appreciate the criminality of one's conduct. Or it may involve adding a volitional as well as cognitive element to the existing standard (e.g., changing the *M'Naghten* standard to the American Law Institute standard).

We also periodically allow the court to consider other mental disabilities that do not rise to the standard of insanity in assessing criminal liability. These are disabilities believed to diminish the defendant's capacity to be fully responsible for a given crime. They are severe enough to justify less punishment than would usually be imposed for that crime, but not so severe as to excuse the defendant altogether. This use of knowledge of psychological incapacity to attenuate the harshness of punishment is referred to as the doctrine of diminished capacity, which includes two variants (Arenella 1977).

Under the so-called *mens rea* variant, defendants can introduce psychological evidence demonstrating that they were disturbed enough at the time of the crime to have lacked full capacity to have one of the elements of the crime with which they are charged. (Note that this doctrine does not necessarily require that defendants actually lack the element of *mens rea*. It merely requires that they have diminished capacity to have one of the criminal elements. This opens the door to broad psychological testimony.) The *mens rea* variant of diminished capacity is used primarily when the law grades the degree of punishment for certain types of conduct and requires different mental elements to be proved at each gradation. Mentally disordered offenders charged with first-degree murder, for example, may contend that they lacked the capacity to premeditate or deliberate. This would reduce their liability to second-degree murder, i.e., killing with intent but without premeditation and deliberation. This approach to diminished capacity was invoked frequently in California in the past two decades and resulted in a number of highly unpopular decisions in which offenders who had committed homicide were given relatively light sentences (Coury 1984). Recently, California abolished its diminished capacity doctrine.

Under the second or so-called partial responsibility variant of the diminished capacity doctrine, defendants can introduce evidence of their disability as formal mitigating factors which, by statute, may shift their offense into a separate category carrying a lower maximum penalty (Walker and McCabe 1973). In England, for example, evidence of a mental impairment at the time a homicide is committed may be utilized to reduce the criminal liability from murder to manslaughter.

Shah (1986) notes that at least 10 states have enacted provisions that follow in large measure the Model Penal Code provision for criminal homicide to be reduced to manslaughter (from murder) when committed under the influence of "extreme mental or emotional disturbance for which there is a reasonable explanation or excuse" (American Law Institute 1980).

The commonest manner in which evidence of psychological differences between offenders is considered in assessing punishment is by modifying the length of the sentence after guilt has been determined. Some jurisdictions are quite liberal in allowing evidence of a defendant's psychological impairments to be heard at a sentencing hearing. The judge or jury may be swayed by such evidence to impose a lesser sentence. (Psychological data also may be used to impose harsher penalties upon offenders if these data suggest they are dangerous.) The recent tendency toward more uniform sentencing is probably diminishing the extent to which courts rely on evidence of psychological variation in determining the length of sentences. The new sentencing schemes (sometimes called presumptive sentencing) do allow for consideration of psychological variations as mitigating or aggravating factors, but they also put strict limits on the range of sentences that can be imposed. Thus, once the defendant is found guilty, even the presence of major psychological infirmities may have little influence in determining the length of his or her sentence (Forer 1980).

Up to now, most efforts to expand consideration of psychological disabilities in assessing liability have had only limited impact on the criminal justice system, and significant change is unlikely in the near future. In our current political climate, pressure is actually growing to avoid examining psychological issues related to culpability by narrowing the insanity defense or doing away with practices associated with the diminished capacity doctrine. Nevertheless, the relentlessness with which efforts to broaden consideration of psychological disabilities have arisen in the past century suggests that our society is hardly unaware of the differences in psychological capacities of defendants. Tension between scientific approaches that emphasize differences among defendants and classical criminological approaches that assume similarities between defendants is always present. It may well be that only the insanity defense keeps that tension at a tolerable level. By providing a loophole for dealing with the worst possible cases, the insanity defense allows society to acknowledge that at least some offenders are different. This enables society to avoid the formidable problems that would arise if it were to adopt a more flexible approach in assessing the relationships of psychological disability to liability in the cases of all offenders.

Knowledge of Mental Disorders and Criminal Responsibility

Evaluations of insanity pose two major problems for clinicians. First, defendants are usually examined some time after the crime has occurred, and their actual psychological state at the time of the crime must be inferred. Second, mental health clinicians do not approach their task armed with a conceptual framework for evaluating the kinds of cognitive and volitional incapacities that are likely to be relevant to the determination of insanity.

Any judgments made concerning a person's mental state at some precise point in what may be the distant past (often months or years) must, as a rule, be based on limited data (Guttmacher and Weihofen 1952). Clinicians try to make these judgments on the basis of their observations regarding the defendant's past history of mental illness and his or her current mental status. Such observations may lead to a diagnosis implying that the defendant at some time in the past suffered from a mental disorder that had a predictable course. It may then be surmised that this particular disorder could have compromised the defendant's capacities at the time of the crime (Goldstein 1967). This hypothesis is bolstered if the description of the defendant's behavior at the time of the crime, or the defendant's recollection of his or her mental status at that time, is compatible with the presence of the type of disorder that has been diagnosed. The process is at best conjectural, and some have questioned whether it is possible to give an expert opinion regarding the defendant's mental state at the time of the crime (Menninger 1968).

The problem of developing a conceptual framework for evaluating a defendant's cognitive and volitional status at the time of the crime requires the clinician to appreciate that what is called for is an evaluation of the defendant's capacities. This is made explicit in the ALI test, which asks whether the defendant lacked substantial capacity to appreciate the criminality of his conduct or to conform his conduct to the requirements of the law. It is implicit, though limited entirely to cognitive elements, in the *M'Naghten* test. Ultimately, any judgment regarding a person's responsibility or blameworthiness can be conceptualized in terms of capacity. When confronted with a situation in which a criminal act is possible, offenders have certain capacities to act in a law-abiding way and to refrain from criminal action. Incapacities that limit the opportunity for noncriminal actions, or that limit the ability to avoid criminal action, can correctly be viewed as influencing the offender's degree of choice and, therefore, his or her responsibility for a given act.

Although clinicians do not usually conceptualize how cognitive and volitional impairments influence a person's capacity to perform an act or to refrain from performing an act, such conceptualization is not beyond their expertise. One way to think about this problem is to hypothesize that offenders make risk/benefit analyses of all possible rewards or punishments society provides for legal or nonlegal behavior and then make the most self-serving responses. It is important to emphasize that this is simply a hypothetical construct. Ordinary offenders are unlikely to go through systematic analyses of the risks and benefits of their conduct.

The benefits of a criminal act can be described as follows:

1. *Gratification of some perceived need.* Sometimes the need is as basic and direct as money, power, or sex. Sometimes the need is more complex. A significant number of crimes are preceded by periods of tension that may in part be alleviated by the performance of a criminal act. The nature of that tension, or its relationship to the criminal act, may be created by motivations that are unconscious or outside of the offender's awareness.

2. *Possibility of peer group support.* Certain types of criminal actions will bring offenders a certain degree of positive reinforcement from individuals whom they depend upon or admire. This is particularly true when offenders are part of a cultural group whose code of moral conduct supports values at variance with those of the greater society.

3. *Increase in self-esteem.* Some offenders have had learning experiences that reinforced them when they behaved in an antisocial manner. As with the second benefit, a social factor is in-

volved. Individuals raised in subcultures that condone criminal activities may feel a greater sense of self-esteem and self-approval when they successfully violate the law.

The risks of committing a criminal act include the following:

1. *Possibility of societal punishment,* usually in the form of imprisonment. The creation of this risk is a major preoccupation of our entire system of correctional justice.

2. *Peer disapproval.* Even if society did not seek to punish offenders, many would consider the possible anger or rejection of other citizens as a major aversive consequence of crime. With or without imprisonment or fine, the moral condemnation of others is substantial punishment, especially when these individuals are closely related to the defendant.

3. *Self-punishment.* To the extent that we are trained to believe that criminal actions are wrongful or bad, and that we are also responsive to such training, the mere anticipation of antisocial behavior elicits an internalized aversive response (i.e., guilt feeling) in most of us. We either punish ourselves more or like ourselves less. It is this particular risk of criminal activity that society hopes will maximize law-abiding behavior and thereby make the other risks of socially imposed punishment or condemnation unnecessary. (For a more complete analysis, it might be useful to delineate the benefits and risks of avoiding an illegal response. The major benefits would be the approval of others and, in particular, self-approval. The major risks would be loss of the gratifications associated with the crime or possible loss of peer or self-approval. But for our purposes here, this analysis is unnecessary.)

Consideration of the foregoing benefits and risks could assist those who must evaluate the relationship of capacity to responsibility if the following three assessments are made:

1. *The degree to which noncriminal and gratifying alternative behaviors were available at the time of the crime.* Usually the perceived needs, conscious or unconscious, that are gratified by committing a crime could also have been gratified in a law-abiding manner. The availability of legal alternatives, however, is often limited by such incapacities as biological deficits, inadequate learning experiences, and lack of particular skills or social discrimination. Those who do not have as many good alternatives as others will exaggerate the benefits of crime. They will be less in-

fluenced by social sanctions than others and may be judged less blameworthy than others. (It should be clear that I am not suggesting that we excuse anyone whose criminality has major sociological determinants. I am just saying that if the poor have fewer alternatives available than the rich, then they may be less blameworthy, particularly for crimes that are motivated by financial gain.)

2. *The extent of the offender's awareness of the benefits and the risks of crime and its alternatives.* It is unlikely that offenders are ever completely aware of all these factors. They will differ in their capacity to perceive, understand, and integrate information related to the criminal act and its consequences. Sometimes, they will be unaware of alternative law-abiding responses. Those who are confused about their purpose in committing an illegal act, or about how others will respond to that act, will be less responsive to societal sanctions and, therefore, less blameworthy than those who have more accurate cognitive and perceptual capacities. This assessment requires an examination of offenders' cognitive and perceptual processes. The presence of any psychiatric disorder that impairs cognition or perception would raise the possibility of diminished blameworthiness.

3. *The offender's capacity to rationally balance the risks and benefits of criminal conduct.* This capacity is powerfully influenced by mental disorders characterized by a tendency to distort the degree of either risk or benefit associated with an act. In some disorders, such as the manic phase of bipolar disorder, individuals may perceive their needs to take certain types of actions as being uncontrollable. For them, the benefits of an action that may subsequently be defined as illegal are greatly exaggerated. Individuals who have anxiety or personality disorders, and who sometimes feel driven to commit illegal acts to reduce states of painful tension, may also exaggerate the benefits of an illegal action. In most psychotic disturbances, the benefits of perceived need, peer group support, or self-approval are likely to be miscalculated. Psychotic illness will also increase the likelihood of poor assessment of the risks of external punishment, social condemnation, or self-condemnation. Depressed offenders may already be subjecting themselves to massive self-punishment. They may not fear societally imposed punishment and may even welcome it. The miscalculation of risk in these individuals can be viewed as an aspect of their inability to comprehend that their depression is not likely to be permanent and that the punishment they will receive is something they will not welcome when they are well.

Any organic brain syndrome will impair the offender's capacities to balance the risks and benefits of a criminal act. Alcohol intoxication, the commonest organic dysfunction at the time of a crime, may be associated with an exaggeration of the benefits of the crime. It is almost always associated with a miscalculation of the risks, insofar as the possibility of external punishment is minimized and the likelihood of future self-punishment is ignored.

An assessment of the availability of alternatives, the degree of awareness of alternatives, the risks and benefits, and the capacity to weigh risks and benefits provides a rough means of judging how individuals may be impaired in their cognitive or volitional capacities. Lack of capacity to perceive or understand information related to the risks and benefits of criminal or noncriminal action will generally relate to cognitive impairment. Defective capacities to utilize noncriminal alternatives or to weigh the risks and benefits of crime will generally relate to volitional impairments.

Legal Controversies Involving the Disposition of Insanity Acquittees

The possibility that insanity acquittees will be set free while still dangerous and, perhaps, commit new crimes has concerned Anglo-American society for many hundreds of years. Although understandable, for the most part this concern has been unwarranted. The most notorious acquittees, whose cases are cited in historical accounts of the insanity defense in England, were all confined to jail or prison immediately following acquittal, and most of them, including Daniel M'Naghten, spent the rest of their lives in confinement (Walker and McCabe 1973). In the United States, the amount of time insanity acquittees have spent in confinement (usually in security hospitals) following acquittal has roughly paralleled the amount of time they would have spent in prison if they had been convicted of the crime for which they were charged (Pasewark 1981). However, as long as the possibility exists that an insanity acquittee might be released prematurely and commit a new crime, many citizens will be concerned that the existence of the insanity defense jeopardizes public safety.

The criminal justice system has responded to this concern by developing mechanisms for ensuring that almost all acquittees will be confined to security hospitals. Legislatures have framed statutes to facilitate the process of committing acquittees to security hospitals for an indeterminate period of time following acquittal. As compared with the process of civil commitment, the commitment of insanity acquittees can be accomplished with relative ease.

All states require a mandatory examination of acquittees to determine if they should be civilly committed. A period of restraint is usually imposed upon the offender until that examination is accomplished (Kerr and Roth in press). Some states, such as Missouri, Delaware, and Kansas, require mandatory indeterminate commitment after acquittal (Morris 1983). In other states, such as Utah and Indiana, acquittees must wait 1 or 2 years before they can even be considered for release. In states that utilize criteria of dangerousness and mental illness for committing either civil patients or acquittees, the dangerousness of acquittees may be assumed from the nature of the crime for which they were charged, while their mental illness may be assumed from the fact that they have successfully invoked the insanity defense (Morris 1983).

Once committed, insanity acquittees have a difficult time obtaining release. Some states, such as California, require that sanity be completely restored before release is possible (California Penal Code 1981). Using this criterion, even offenders who are no longer viewed as dangerous can be restrained. Other states, such as Delaware, will continue to restrain offenders who are no longer insane but who are still viewed as dangerous (Delaware Code Ann. 1979). Thus, offenders viewed as unsafe or insane may be retained. This contrasts with criteria for the release of those civilly committed who are ordinarily released if they are either "safe" or "sane."

Procedural handicaps also are placed on insanity acquittees who seek release. Unlike civilly committed patients, in many jurisdictions they cannot be released when their psychiatrists or hospital superintendents conclude they no longer need hospitalization (German and Singer 1976). The court may retain control over release and may overrule a doctor's recommendation. Some states, such as Kansas, require the prosecutor or district attorney who tried the acquittee's original case to participate in any release hearing initiated by the acquittee (Kansas Stat. Ann. 1980). The court also regulates issues such as receiving passes to go out of the secure setting, the degree of security imposed upon them, and conditional release (Morris 1983). Finally, unlike persons civilly committed, they are not always entitled to periodic judicial review of their confinement (German and Singer 1976).

The logic justifying practices that make it easy to restrain and difficult to release insanity acquittees is not always apparent. Even though it may be assumed that defendants would not actually have pleaded insanity unless they had committed the act with which they have been charged, acquittees are technically "not guilty." The automatic inference that they are dangerous may not be justified, particularly when the crimes they were charged with were not crimes of violence. Nor is it necessarily true that, if they were dangerous at the time they committed the criminal act, they are still dangerous at the time of acquittal. Many months may have elapsed between the crime and the acquittal, and the assumption that dangerous tendencies have not abated during this time may be inaccurate.

The question also arises whether the insanity acquittee is sufficiently mentally ill as to need continued hospital treatment. In some jurisdictions, the insanity of acquittees is never proven at the time of trial. Only a reasonable doubt is cast upon their sanity. (This occurs in jurisdictions in which all of the elements of a crime, including the defendant's sanity, must be proved by the prosecution beyond a reasonable doubt.) Furthermore, there is always reason to suspect that the defendant's psychological condition at the time of acquittal is better than it was at the time of the crime. As noted previously, in order to go to trial the defendant must be found competent to stand trial. Such a finding assumes at least some degree of mental stability and provides a rationale for questioning the continuing presumption of mental illness.

In the civil libertarian climate of the late 1960s and 1970s, many of the assumptions regarding the alleged dangerousness and mental illness of insanity acquittees began to be questioned by the courts. In a series of court rulings, the laws of states, such as Michigan and New Jersey, which provided for automatic indeterminate commitment of insanity acquittees, were found to be in violation of the Equal Protection and Due Process requirements of the Constitution (*People v. McQuillan* 1974; *State v. Krol* 1975). The courts rejected the idea that the state could use commitment standards and procedures for insanity acquittees that were markedly different from those used for civil commitment. They ruled that, following acquittal, these individuals had a right to a new hearing at which confinement to a security hospital was possible only if they met the criteria of civil commitment—namely, current dangerousness and mental illness. Using these criteria, a significant number of insanity acquittees were able to avoid continued restraint. In the year following the *McQuillan* decision in Michigan, more than 60 acquittees were released after a civil hearing determining that they did not meet the criteria of civil commitment (Schwartz 1975).

The release of a significant number of persons who were suspected of being guilty of a variety of serious crimes was unprecedented in the State of Michigan and aroused a great deal of public concern. Levels of indignation soared when two insanity acquittees committed particularly violent crimes shortly after their release. Understandably, a powerful public outcry emerged at this point for greater control over insanity acquittees. One response was the passing of a so-called "guilty but mentally ill" statute (to be discussed later), which provides the jury with the option of convicting and sentencing those who plead insanity and providing them with some form of treatment. As of this writing, 10 states have passed "guilty but mentally ill" statutes somewhat similar to that of Michigan (viz., Alaska, Delaware, Georgia, Indiana, Illinois, Kentucky, New Mexico, Pennsylvania, South Dakota, and Utah). Another response was an increased demand that insanity acquittees charged with violent offenses be treated differently than those civilly committed, and that they be subjected to greater control and monitoring in their efforts to be released to the community (Bloom and Bloom 1981).

It appears that, even before the Hinckley case, the pendulum had begun to shift away from a less restrictive to a more controlling approach to the insanity acquittee. In June 1983, the restrictive trend was significantly strengthened by the Supreme Court. The petitioner in *Jones v. United States* 1983) spent several years at St. Elizabeths Hospital following acquittal by reason of insanity for a misdemeanor that carried a maximum sentence of 1 year. Jones contended that he was denied the procedural protections usually provided in civil commitment, and that even if the court recognized a legitimate justification for the automatic commitment of insanity acquittees, such justification was insufficient after an acquittee had been confined for as long as would have been possible had he been convicted of the offense charged. The Court rejected both arguments and made the following rulings:

1. That Jones' acquittal by reason of insanity entailed a finding beyond a reasonable doubt that Jones had committed an illegal act;
2. That this finding "certainly indicates dangerousness";
3. That it is not unreasonable to infer that someone who is insane at the time of an offense continues to be mentally ill after his trial; and

4. That no correlation exists between the severity of the offense
and the time needed for treatment and recovery. The Court
noted that "the length of the acquittee's hypothetical criminal
sentence, therefore, is irrelevant to the purpose of his confinement" (*Jones v. United States* 1983).

The Jones decision thus allows states to use existing statutes, or
to draft new ones, that substantially diminish the opportunity of
acquittees to gain freedom, irrespective of their mental status.
How much of the Court's response was influenced by the furor
following the Hinckley acquittal is unclear, but its message is
clear. It is constitutionally permissible for states to provide for indeterminate confinement following a finding of not guilty by reason of insanity, in consideration of public safety. The great majority of insanity acquittees will, as in the pre-civil-libertarian
era, continue to be restrained or monitored by the criminal justice
system.

Clinical Issues

Mental Health Skills Used in Assessing Responsibility

Although many comments can be found in the legal literature
to the effect that mental health professionals have no training or
experience in assessing criminal responsibility, a brief look at the
nature of clinical practice suggests that this is not entirely true.
The assessment of responsibility is, in fact, a routine part of many
aspects of medical practice. Such assessment is also required in
most forms of psychotherapy or counseling. Physicians must regularly communicate judgments to patients regarding which symptoms or behaviors will be excused and which will not. When doctors treat patients with severe physical disabilities, they do not
(with a few exceptions) hold them responsible for having developed their disease. Skilled doctors, however, do not excuse all
symptoms or behavior. Often, they invoke the concept of responsibility in order to elicit maximum cooperation from patients.

Even when the physically ill are not held accountable for developing their illness, they are usually held accountable for what
they do about it. Patients who have just had heart attacks will be
told that their survival is in their hands—that if they have the
will to change their lifestyle, they will live longer. Similar mes-
sages are given to alcoholics. In effect, alcoholics are treated as
though they are afflicted with a disease for which they are not

responsible. At the same time, these "afflicted" patients are held fully responsible for taking the first drink that brings on the dire consequences of alcoholism.

In dealing with mental disorders, depressed patients are treated in a manner that does not push them beyond their capacities. They may be told at times that it would be useful for them to accept the idea that there is very little they can do to control their underlying illness. Even severely depressed patients, however, may be asked to take responsibility for things they can control, such as cooperating with the treatment regimen or participating in various aspects of therapy.

In the process of psychotherapy, mental health clinicians try to help patients feel less intrapunitive or responsible for past misconduct by helping them understand the forces that determined it. Patients are provided with explanations of past behavior that imply that they were not fully responsible for what they did. At the same time, however, therapists usually hold their patients fully responsible for everything that happens once psychotherapy is started (Halleck 1984). Sometimes, therapists phrase their ascription of responsibility in terms of the concept of choice. They will disapprove of any behavior that obstructs the process of therapy and will refer to it in such pejorative terms as "resistance" or "acting out." Patients are told that they are choosing to be obstructive and that they can choose to be more cooperative. (Physicians also ascribe responsibility in terms of choice. A post-coronary patient who overeats, drinks, or smokes will be blamed for "choosing" self-harmful activities and for failing to "choose" desirable activities, such as exercise.)

Although the assessment of responsibility is a daily task for mental health clinicians, crucial differences characterize how this task is approached in the clinical setting and how it must be performed in the courtroom. In clinical practice, the techniques clinicians use to excuse or to assess blame are, with rare exceptions, developed for the sole purpose of helping the patient. They have a utilitarian rather than a moral objective. When punishment is invoked, it is the minimum required to shape behavior. As a rule, the most severe punishments clinicians provide are disapproval or withdrawal. Because severe punishment is not at issue, mental health clinicians in ordinary clinical practice can be relatively relaxed in making assessments of responsibility. The consequences of too much, too little, or inconsistent blaming are unlikely to be overly harmful unless the faulty assessments are repeated many times. This situation contrasts with the grim consequences of ascription of responsibility in the criminal justice system, where severe punishment is common and may have powerful consequences for the offender.

Dangers of Intuitive Conceptualization of Responsibility

Although mental health professionals regularly deal with the issue of responsibility, they do not, as a rule, conceptualize the manner in which they go about assessing it. The only clinicians who regularly consider the issue of responsibility as it relates to psychotherapy or psychiatric treatment are attribution theorists, who believe that the manner in which people perceive the causation of their behavior is an important variable in determining behavioral change (Strong 1978). Clinicians are prone to ascribe blame on the basis of clinical experience or intuition. Since their own views of responsibility (like everyone else's) are likely to reflect their previously learned values, two clinicians, both of whom use an intuitive approach, cannot be expected to consistently come up with the same conclusions. The manner in which clinicians have learned to assess blame in the course of their clinical training may also influence their view of responsibility. Psychoanalytically oriented clinicians, who are trained to view past experiences as determining present behavior, may be more generous excusers than biologically oriented clinicians, who may be reluctant to excuse unless a physical defect is apparent.

To the extent that clinicians fail to conceptualize the manner in which they ascribe responsibility, their testimony in criminal insanity cases may be confusing to the jury. In responding to the M'Naghten or ALI tests of insanity, clinicians are actually making a statement as to the defendant's responsibility. Unless clinical experts can clearly define the reasons why they believe an individual is blameworthy or not, jurors will be unable to determine how much of their opinion is based on personal values as opposed to professional knowledge.

As noted in an earlier section, I believe that clinicians are most valuable to the courts when they conceptualize their assessments of responsibility in terms of the defendant's capacities. An offender's capacities to refrain from a criminal act or to behave in a law-abiding manner can be assessed in terms of awareness of the availability of alternatives, awareness of risks and benefits, and ability to weigh risks and benefits. Clinicians can describe impairments of these qualities in terms that are relatively free of jargon and understandable to jurors. Such testimony is far preferable to conclusory statements that an individual does or does not meet the requirements of the *M'Naghten* or ALI standards. The assessment of criminal responsibility can, of course, never be value-free, but if it is conceptualized in terms of capacities, it can at least be discussed in rational rather than mystical terms.

When to Recommend Release

It is always difficult to determine when an individual who has a history of violent or antisocial behavior can be safely released from a hospital setting, and some of the general issues involved in making such decisions will be discussed in the next chapter. The release of insanity acquittees, however, poses some special problems, which will be briefly noted here. Presumably, the crimes of those acquitted by reason of insanity were in large part caused by their mental illness. Successful treatment of such an illness should, in theory, diminish the dangerousness of acquittees. Some discouraging data, however, suggest that released insanity acquittees commit new crimes at about the same rate as released felons who were imprisoned for the same type of crimes (Pasewark 1981). This suggests either that treatment is ineffective or that the criminality of some insanity acquittees may be determined by factors in addition to, or independent of, the mental illness that is believed to have engendered their insanity.

While systematic studies of the nature of the mental disorders characterizing insanity acquittees are lacking, some reason exists to suspect that the nature of their disorders differs significantly from that found in ordinary mental patients who are not usually violent (Rabkin 1979; Steadman and Braff 1983). Experienced clinicians believe that insanity acquittees can often be characterized by mixed diagnoses, with some symptoms of psychosis and some of severe personality disorders. (As a rule, it is the presence of psychosis that leads to a finding of insanity. The presence of a personality disorder is most likely to be associated with criminal tendencies. An appreciation of the mixed disorders found among acquittees may explain the high recidivism rate of those who are released and alert clinicians to special problems of treatment.)

In the majority of instances, treatment of acquittees is focused on their psychosis. Their personality disorders are not treated, either because they are believed to be untreatable or because skills or facilities for providing such treatment are lacking. As a consequence, offenders successfully treated for psychosis may still retain personality characteristics associated with criminality. Their criminal propensities may be better controlled when the psychosis is in remission, but they may not be entirely absent. Even minor subsequent change in the offender's psychological or sociological status may be sufficient to elicit new antisocial behavior. This is an especially difficult problem with acquittees whose psychosis has been controlled with medication and who are then released. The risk of their committing new crimes is high if they stop taking their medication.

Some insanity acquittees have obvious psychotic disorders that are treatable and are not associated with other disorders. Clinicians can usually recommend release of these offenders when their psychosis is adequately treated. However, where symptoms of certain personality disorders (particularly paranoid, antisocial, narcissistic, and borderline disorders) are prominent aspects of the acquittees' past and current behavior, clinicians must exercise great caution in recommending release, as well as prudently advise that such acquittees receive continued treatment and supervision in the community.

Emerging Legal Trends

Controlling the Diversion of Insane Offenders

As in the case of the incompetency diversion, legal trends related to the insanity defense will reflect a tension between public demand for safety and concern with the rights of offenders. Following the acquittal on grounds of insanity of the attempted Presidential assassin John Hinckley, Jr., the policy trend has certainly been toward providing greater public protection. Some of the recent proposals for changes in the insanity trial and in the disposition of acquittees have already been discussed but will be noted again in this section. Two approaches are available to increase the certainty that insanity acquittees will not go free. The most direct strategy is to restrict the number of insanity acquittals. A second strategy is to strengthen controls on those who are so acquitted.

Reducing Acquittals

The most extreme proposal for reducing the number of acquittals is to abolish the insanity defense. It is important to note that abolishment will not totally eliminate the consideration of mental disability in determining liability. To find guilt, the state must still prove that defendants possessed the required *mens rea* for the particular crime charged. In most jurisdictions, however, the *mens rea* is defined in such a way that evidence of the defendant's mental illness will not negate it unless there is extraordinarily severe cognitive impairment.

Other proposals have recently been made to tighten the standards by which exculpatory insanity is determined. These rely primarily on some variation of the *M'Naghten* standard, which excuses only on the basis of severe cognitive impairment, rather than on the American Law Institute standard, which excuses for either cognitive or volitional impairment. Awareness is growing among both attorneys and psychiatrists that the concept of volition, whether framed in terms of irresistible impulse or inability to conform one's conduct to the requirements of the law, is a murky one and susceptible to circular reasoning (Halleck 1984). No scientific way is known to determine when an impulse is uncontrollable and when it is simply not controlled. Too often, statements that individuals cannot control their behavior are simply judgments that they should not be blamed for what they have done.

Proposals have also been made to place the burden of proving insanity upon the defendant in all jurisdictions (American Psychiatric Association 1982). In the Hinckley case, the prosecution had to prove beyond a reasonable doubt that the defendant was sane. This was no small task when the defendant had committed a crime for bizarre reasons. Putting the burden of proving insanity upon the defendant is likely to reduce the number of insanity acquittals in those jurisdictions that currently place the burden of proving sanity on the prosecution.

The Hinckley case has also encouraged legislators and attorneys to take a more careful look at the nature of psychiatric testimony. Concern is increasing that conclusory testimony usurps the function of the jury and provides mental health expert witnesses with too much power in influencing the jury. Legislators fear that defense experts are especially prone to abuse this power to gain acquittals. Psychiatrists are themselves concerned that testifying in a conclusory manner reinforces the public's misconception of psychiatry, creates what is often an illusory battle of the experts, and generally contributes to the deterioration of the image of the psychiatric profession (American Psychiatric Association 1982). And, as noted earlier, the Federal Comprehensive Crime Control Act of 1984 limits the scope of expert testimony on the ultimate legal issues that are to be determined by the triers of fact, viz., the jury and judge. If a substantial number of states follow this policy, an interesting spillover could occur with regard to modifying the use of conclusory expert testimony in other areas, such as competency or dangerousness.

We are also likely to see continuing efforts to modify the use of the doctrines of diminished capacity or diminished responsibility in determining the degree of punishment inflicted upon the defender. California has recently abolished its rather idiosyncratic interpretation of the mental elements of "premeditation" and "malice," which, in the past, allowed mental health experts considerable leeway in testifying that psychological disturbances limited the defendant's capacity to have the requisite *mens rea* in cases of first- or second-degree murder. Few states seem eager to repeat the California experiment. However, use of the diminished capacity doctrine will probably decrease unless, as noted above, states that have abolished the insanity defense turn to this doctrine as the only means of providing mercy.

If attempts at abolition or creation of stricter standards and procedures for determining insanity result in fewer insanity acquittals, it is reasonable to ask what will happen when those who were once diverted are now sent to prison. The most likely prediction is that the impact of such a change would be negligible. Many seriously disordered offenders are already in prison. Nevertheless, raising the size of this population by even a small increment may bring on new calls for better mental health services in prisons. But even such a limited change is unlikely in a period of great budgetary restraint.

The "Guilty But Mentally Ill" Alternative

The Hinckley acquittal also seems to have increased the popularity of the "guilty but mentally ill" (GBMI) alternative. In several states, juries now have an alternative verdict to the traditional verdicts of guilty, not guilty, or not guilty by reason of insanity. They are given the option of finding defendants who have raised the insanity defense "guilty but mentally ill." Those adjudicated GBMI are formally recognized as different from the ordinary offender. At the same time, they are sentenced under ordinary criminal codes and can be given a lengthy sentence. Recognition of the special status of these offenders is accompanied by a requirement that, once sentenced, they receive some type of mental health treatment while serving their prison term. The GBMI plea gives the jury an opportunity to recognize that some defendants have severe enough disorders to be categorized differently from other defendants, while at the same time ensuring that these defendants are not set free.

Unfortunately, the GBMI alternative gives the jury an easy way out of grappling with the more difficult moral issues inherent in adjudicating guilt or innocence. It has been criticized, therefore, as diluting the moral power of the insanity defense (American Psychiatric Association 1982). If the jury can avoid deciding who is not liable as a result of mental illness, there may be too few exceptions to prove the rule that the overwhelming majority of offenders are sane. The certainty that those who are convicted are actually culpable may become a little more doubtful.

The GBMI alternative is best viewed as a device for reducing the number of insanity acquittals. It is especially popular with prosecutors who believe that some jurors who might be reluctant to find mentally disordered defendants guilty, and who might lean toward acquittal on the basis of insanity, can be convinced that the GBMI verdict is a just compromise. The state effectively obtains a conviction, while the jury believes it has provided the offender with a humane and compassionate disposition and avoids the moral task of deciding which offender should be excused. Actually, little reason exists to believe that offenders sentenced as GBMI will in fact be treated differently than ordinary offenders. Mental health treatment has, in theory, always been available to those found guilty and sentenced to prisons. The GBMI alternative offers no new advantages to offenders (and can hardly be distinguished from an ordinary criminal conviction), unless it is accompanied by a firm commitment on the part of the state to expand its treatment resources and provide offenders with adequate mental health treatment. So far, no evidence shows that this is happening (Grostic 1978).

Restraining Insanity Acquittees

While the trend toward imposing increased restraints on acquittees has been strengthened following the Hinckley acquittal and the *Jones* decision, it still remains unclear how the states will eventually shape their release policies. The following issues are likely to receive increasing attention:

1. Should special legislation allowing for easier commitment and detention of acquittees be created for all acquittees or only for those charged with violent crimes?
2. Should the nature of the institutions to which the acquittees are

sent be determined by the court, by the legislature, or by the treating agencies?

3. How frequently should the acquittee be entitled to a judicial review of his or her confinement?
4. Should the eventual release of the acquittee be determined by the institution, by the committing court, or by a special review board akin to a parole board?
5. What role should mental health professionals play either in recommending retention or release or in being members of review boards that govern release?
6. How can a system of conditional release be developed so that the activities of acquittees released to the community can carefully be monitored and their participation in treatment ensured?
7. Should the insanity acquittee who is unresponsive to treatment but remains dangerous continue to be confined in a hospital rather than a prison?
8. What should be done with the acquittee who is unresponsive to treatment but, for such reasons as aging or infirmity, is no longer likely to be dangerous?

Perhaps the most critical of these questions are those dealing with possession of the ultimate power to determine the timing and circumstances of releasing acquittees to the community. One model (currently in use in Oregon) that is likely to be especially appealing involves delegating such authority to several individuals who constitute a special review board (Rogers 1982). This approach allows the interests of various groups to be represented in any release decision. It also makes available resources for postrelease monitoring and care and diffuses responsibility for decisions to release offenders who subsequently may be violent. This diffusion may help clinicians avoid malpractice suits for negligent release.

CHAPTER 5

Special Sentencing and Treatment for Mentally Disordered Offenders Viewed as Dangerous

THROUGHOUT MOST OF THIS CENTURY, those who administer the criminal justice system have retained the belief that a few offenders are abnormal individuals who have a particularly high risk of repeating their crimes, and that they can be prevented from doing so if they are properly treated. These individuals are felt to be both mentally disordered and dangerous and also in need of special care, either within a prison or in a security hospital. It is assumed that merely sentencing them to a correctional setting will not help to change their behavior and, in the long run, will not serve the purpose of protecting society. Here, the concern of the criminal justice system is not with the offender's mental condition at the time of the crime or the time of the trial but rather with a preexisting mental disorder that is assumed to be chronic and to increase the likelihood that the offender will harm society at some time in the future. The judicial decision to divert such offenders to specialized treatment programs is generally made only after they have been convicted.

Identification and Disposition of Dangerous Offenders

Who is Diverted and Why?

At various times over the past 40 years, different states have experimented with programs requiring specialized disposition for offenders believed to be mentally disordered or mentally retarded and dangerous to society. Specialized disposition usually requires involuntary commitment to a treatment program for an indefinite

period of time. Most of these programs were created to treat offenders who committed sex-related crimes, but some focused on
specialized treatment of other classes of allegedly dangerous offenders who were usually referred to as "defective delinquents"
(Dix 1983).

The term "defective delinquent" is unfortunate insofar as it
seems to imply that those who are diverted are mentally retarded.
The first defective delinquent program, developed in Massachusetts in 1911, did deal with mentally retarded offenders. Subsequently, however, the term "defective delinquent" began to be
used to identify disruptive, recidivistic offenders who were
believed to have mental abnormalities and who seemed to be unresponsive to rehabilitation in the ordinary prison setting (Boslow
and Kohlmeyer 1963). Some who qualified for this disposition
were mentally retarded, but most were not. The most carefully
implemented and studied of these programs was created by the
Maryland Defective Delinquency statute in 1951. In the 1940s and
1950s, indeterminate treatment programs, especially those designed
to identify and treat the so-called sexual psychopath, were extremely popular (Sutherland 1950). By 1959, fully 27 states and
the District of Columbia had such laws (American Bar Association
1984).

In recent years, those defective delinquency programs that dealt
with nonsexual offenders have either been terminated or substantially modified, so that, for the most part, they now provide treatment on a voluntary basis only. Offenders sent to those programs
still in operation are no longer institutionalized indefinitely but
are discharged at the expiration of their criminal sentences (Kohlmeyer 1979). Indeterminate sex offender programs have also lost
popularity and have been disappearing rapidly. Currently, only
five states have a provision allowing for indefinite commitment of
sexual psychopaths (American Bar Association 1984). Moreover,
several groups, including the American Bar Association's Criminal
Justice Mental Health Standards, have called for the repeal of sexual psychopath statutes.

Throughout this chapter, offenders who are given specialized
dispositions following conviction, including some type of indeterminate sentencing and treatment, will be referred to as mentally disordered sex offenders. For practical purposes, sex offenders constitute the only group who are currently subject to this
form of disposition. One exception to this statement exists in
Kansas, where convicted offenders of any type may be sent to a
mental health facility if a psychiatric examination reveals that

they are in need of treatment and such a commitment is not likely to endanger either society or the defendant (Dix 1983).

A major societal objective in creating specialized treatment programs for mentally disordered sex offenders is that of protecting the public. Another objective may be a wish to help the offender. When efforts are made to treat the emotional problems of sex offenders, however, the provision of help is based primarily on societal needs rather than those of the offender. It is assumed that, if sex offenders are successfully treated, the public will be safer when they are eventually released. The statutes that created those sex offender programs still in existence were often drafted after the occurrence of some particularly heinous and well-publicized sex crime. Legislators hoped that the indeterminate aspects of the programs would appease the public outcry for more protection, while the treatment aspect would ensure that offenders received the most "enlightened" and "scientific" interventions available (Guttmacher and Weihofen 1952).

It is not entirely clear why sex offenders have been singled out for special concern. Certainly, the issue of specialized treatment is never raised for many violent offenders who commit nonsexual crimes. One possibility is the prevailing societal belief that those who have sexually deviant motivations are especially dangerous, because they have reduced capacity to control their behavior. Society has ample opportunity to observe that even sexual behavior viewed as normal is not easily controlled by social sanctions. It is easy then to assume that deviant sexual activities, which often appear to be bizarre, and which are expressed even at the risk of severe punishment, are extremely difficult to resist. This view of deviant sexuality is supported by mental health professionals, who consider such conduct to be evidence of mental disorders (American Psychiatric Association 1980). In effect, society treats selected sexually deviant persons as though they have volitional impairments. Such impairments are not considered severe enough to qualify the sex offender for an insanity defense or any other exculpatory advantage, but rather are used to justify greater restraint and, perhaps, treatment.

Duration and Locus of Treatment

Sex offender statutes call for treatment programs based on some degree of indeterminate sentencing. In some states, defendants committed to such programs can, in theory, spend the rest of their lives in a custodial setting. Other programs provide an indeterminate minimum sentence (offenders can be released whenever "cured") but a determinate maximum sentence (offenders cannot be restrained beyond the maximum limits of their sentencing).

A recent survey indicated that in 1978 mentally disordered sex offenders made up 6 percent of all admissions to security hospitals, and constituted 17 percent of the population of formally designated mentally disordered offenders residing in those hospitals. On the average, these offenders remained confined for a little over 2 years (Monahan and Davis 1983).

The actual number of formally designated mentally disordered sex offenders may be considerably larger than the foregoing figures suggest. Many are likely to be treated in other settings. A few mentally disordered sex offenders are put on probation or parole and treated as outpatients. Others are treated in public mental hospitals on either a voluntary or involuntary basis. Still others are committed to specialized programs but are housed in ordinary prisons. They are treated differently than other offenders only with regard to the relative indeterminacy of their sentences and the requirement that their release is in part contingent on participation in some type of treatment program.

Many sex offenders in prison are not formally adjudicated as mentally disordered sex offenders. One prison psychologist has observed that, in five states surveyed, 25 to 30 percent of incarcerated inmates were actually sex offenders (Groth 1982). Some of these persons are imprisoned in states that do not have sex offender statutes. They are sentenced as ordinary offenders (i.e., they are given fixed sentences) but are likely to volunteer for treatment once in prison. As a rule, sex offenders receive more treatment in prison than other offenders even when they have no special designation. This is only partly because they perceive their sexual behavior as "sick" and volunteer for treatment. Mental health professionals who work in prisons tend to view these offenders as mentally disturbed and often try to persuade them to enter therapy (Groth 1979).

Other Issues Related to Identification and Disposition

States that still operate formal programs for the treatment of mentally disordered sex offenders have varied procedures for identifying them. Usually the examination is triggered when the offender is convicted of an offense that is believed to be sexually motivated. Depending on the jurisdiction, the prosecutor, the judge, or the defense attorney may request an evaluation. An estimated 3,600 such evaluations were performed in 1978 (Monahan and Davis 1983). Evaluations are usually conducted by psychiatrists or psychologists in community jails, in outpatient settings, or in security hospitals. In all states, offenders are given a judicial hearing in which the decision to sentence them to a specialized program is made.

Statutes differ in the criteria required to determine need for special treatment. Some states emphasize the requirement of a mental disorder or impairment. The type of disorder is usually not specified, except to note that it must be associated with or be the cause of dangerous behavior. Only a small number of those committed as mentally disordered sex offenders are psychotic. Most are diagnosed as having a personality disorder. Often, the sex crime itself appears to determine the diagnosis. Certain patterns of sexual deviancy are part of the criteria for a group of disorders formally listed as Psychosexual Disorders in the third edition of the American Psychiatric Association's *Diagnostic and Statistical Manual of Mental Disorders* (DSM-III; American Psychiatric Association 1980). An individual who repeatedly engages in these deviant behaviors may be automatically assumed to be mentally disordered.

Since dangerousness is not always defined by statute, it is usually inferred from the seriousness of the sex crime and the frequency with which it has been repeated. The statutes of Massachusetts and Oregon are representative.

In Massachusetts, a "sexually dangerous person" is

any person whose misconduct in sexual matters indicates a general lack of power to control his sexual impulses, as evidenced by repetitive or compulsive behavior and either violence or aggression by an adult against a victim under the age of 16 years, and who as a result is likely to attack or otherwise inflict injury on the objects of his uncontrolled or uncontrollable desires. (Mass. Ann. Laws, Chapter 123A, Section 1, 1982 Supplement)

In Oregon, a "sexually dangerous person" is one

who because of repeated or compulsive acts of misconduct in sexual matters, or because of mental disease or defect, is deemed as likely to continue such acts and to be a danger to others persons. (Oregon Rev. Statutes, Section 426.510, 1981)

In practice, individuals who have raped or attempted to rape adults or molested young children on more than one occasion are almost certain to be viewed as dangerous sex offenders. More controversy exists over crimes involving sexual activity with minor adolescents and exhibitionism. Although these crimes tend to be repetitive, it is unclear how much harm they inflict upon victims. Some statutes also have provisions for a specialized disposition for persons who commit crimes such as arson, which may at times be motivated by sexual drives. In past years, when belief in the efficacy of treatment of sex offenders was greater, many statutes required some evidence that offenders were in need of treatment or likely to benefit from it. These days, only a few statutes require treatability as a condition for a specialized disposition.

Once diverted to a specialized treatment program, mentally disordered sex offenders usually receive some type of treatment; their release is determined by a judicial agency, often the court that recommended the special disposition. Those actually responsible for treatment may have only a limited role in the discharge process. As a rule, the superintendent of the institution where the treatment was conducted must initiate the proceedings by petitioning for the offenders' release. The court or an official review board must then decide whether release is indicated or justified. The releasing agency usually has a number of options in planning release, including the use of parole and home visits.

Legal Issues

The number of mentally disordered sex offenders who are formally adjudicated as needing specialized treatment may be diminishing, but the issues involved in their diversion are broad and raise basic questions about the management of the criminal justice system. Specialized treatment programs call attention to critical legal issues, such as defining dangerousness, the use of indeterminate sentencing, and the manner in which psychological factors are to be considered in the sentencing and release process. Participation in specialized treatment programs also encourages clinicians to focus special attention to conceptualize the problem of predicting dangerousness in sentencing and release decisions, and also to define and acknowledge the extent and limits of their predictive capabilities.

Defining Dangerousness

The term "dangerousness" tends to be defined loosely, both in statutes and in case law. In large part, the difficult task of precise definition has been left to academicians and researchers. Thus, it has been noted that danger implies a relationship in which one person is exposed to harm by another (Sarbin 1967). According to Brooks (1974), the term "dangerousness" can be broken down into at least four component elements: (1) magnitude of harm, (2) probability that the harm will occur, (3) frequency with which the harm will occur, and (4) imminence of the harm. A person can be characterized as "dangerous" or not, depending on how these four components are balanced. For example,

> a harm which is not likely to occur but which is very serious may add up to dangerousness. By the same token a relatively trivial harm which is highly likely to occur with great frequency might also add up to dangerousness. On the other hand a trivial harm even though it is likely to occur, might not add up to dangerousness. (Brooks 1974)

Brooks goes on to note that calling a person "dangerous" is expressing a judgment in the form of a prediction about that individual's future behavior. It is the potentiality for harmfulness that defines dangerousness. Other scholars who have focused on the process of predicting dangerousness have narrowed their attention to the occurrence of violent acts (Shah 1978; Monahan 1981). Violence is defined as acts that involve overt or threatened force and that are likely to result in physical injury to people (Megargee 1976). Forceful acts may also be viewed as violent if they result in great psychological harm. Definitions involving force do not include all possible harms to persons. They do not cover conduct such as child molestation, which is usually considered a form of violence but which creates harm without involving force. Nor do such definitions take into consideration crimes of omission or negligence, which may ultimately inflict enormous physical harm upon people without the use of force.

Those who struggle to define violence or dangerousness come to appreciate that no definition of either term can be precise nor completely free of moral or political judgments. The use of force in a cause viewed as worthy is not usually defined as violence and is unlikely to be seen as dangerous. On the other hand, we consider certain forms of nonforceful dissent as violent acts if they threaten the stability of institutions in which we believe. The degree to which harm caused by neglect is viewed as dangerous will vary with the conscience of the community. Currently, we are deeply preoccupied with child neglect and drunken driving. Throughout much of our recent history, however, we have paid much less attention to the harmfulness of such conduct. Crimes of negligence committed by corporate executives that result in defective products, by government inspectors who allow dangerous workplace conditions to remain uncorrected, or by business people who dispose of waste products indiscriminately may harm many more people than are harmed by street crime (Reiman 1979). Yet, society does not consider such crimes to be nearly as dangerous as street crime.

In defining dangerousness, it is also important to exercise care in determining how this quality will be ascribed to individuals. If individuals have committed acts that have harmed others, we can say with some certainty that they have been dangerous. But society finds limited value in describing dangerousness on the basis of past behavior. Society is interested in future conduct, in predicting which individuals will cause harm. Those who have struggled with the problem of predicting dangerousness have learned that the best that anyone can do, given our current level of knowledge, is to predict a certain probability that a particular event will occur. When one individual is said to be more dangerous than others, the statement simply means that such a person is more likely to commit a particular harmful act in a given timeframe and under certain circumstances. The dangerousness of a given individual is not a fixed trait, but a degree of potentiality to engage in a particular type of behavior, which is likely to change over time (Shah 1978).

To make matters even more complicated, statutes that provide guidelines for determining dangerousness never state what level of probability for what type of harm will constitute dangerousness. Such judgments must be made by the courts or mental health experts on a case-by-case basis. The value systems of juries and clinicians, as well as society's changing perceptions of the harmfulness of various behaviors, will ultimately have considerable influence on what behaviors or potentialities are called dangerous. The vagueness of our statutes either may reflect the unwillingness of lawmakers to deal with the complexities of the definitional problem, or it may simply be a manifestation of their wish to ensure that assessments of dangerousness reflect the prevailing morality of the community. Since dangerousness is such a vague and complex concept, certain virtues may be found in not defining it too carefully and allowing the court or other judicial agencies, functioning as the conscience of the community, considerable leeway in deciding whom they will so designate.

Despite all the noted difficulties, society still has a powerful need to try to predict the occurrence of behavior it views as dangerous. To the extent that it can make accurate predictions, it can take preventive measures that may increase public safety. Shah has listed 15 points in the legal and mental health systems at which estimates of future harmful conduct are made (Shah 1978). Many of these evaluations involve mentally disordered offenders and are required by statute.

Predicting Dangerousness

Even when defined specifically as violence, dangerousness is difficult to predict accurately. Few situations exist in which any predictor can foresee a 100-percent or even a 50-percent chance that a dangerous act will occur within a given timeframe. Violent acts are relatively infrequent events, and even when an offender has a strong propensity toward committing them, they are not very likely to happen (Meehl 1973). This is because violent acts are determined by many unpredictable circumstances, such as the availability and behavior of victims, access to weapons, changes in the offender's immediate psychological or social status, or interventions on the part of other parties.

Given the limited accuracy of prediction and the grave consequences of a failure to predict violence, a natural tendency among those responsible for dealing with offenders leads them to overpredict violence. Mental health professionals are no exception. Psychiatrists are particularly likely to overpredict dangerousness, because as physicians they have been trained to overpredict serious outcomes. Predicting that a patient who is mildly nervous and depressed may have a brain tumor may seem farfetched, but even if the prediction is wrong it will only require the patient to take more tests and be inconvenienced. The patient may even be reassured by the doctor's thoroughness. On the other hand, doctors receive substantial negative consequences from their patients, their colleagues, society, and themselves when they fail to predict, and thereby fail to discover, a potentially lethal condition. Unfortunately, the consequences of overprediction in the criminal justice system, which often include lengthy incarceration, are quite drastic for the offender. Also, less corrective feedback of overprediction is received in dealing with offenders than in ordinary clinical practice. Physicians learn about their false positive predictions in ordinary practice when the predicted serious outcome does not materialize. If, however, as a result of predicting violence offenders are restrained for a significant period of time, mental health professionals may never learn about the inaccuracy of their predictions.

Whether they have been oblivious to the differences between predicting violent behavior in the criminal justice system and predicting illness in patients, or whether they actually believed they had sufficient skills to determine who would be violent, it must be acknowledged that throughout most of this century many psychiatrists (as well as other mental health professionals) have willingly assumed the task of predicting violence. Society has been eager to delegate this function to them and has seemed to have faith in their skills. In the 1960s and 1970s, however, a growing awareness of the dangers of overprediction, supported by studies demonstrating that mental health professionals could not accurately predict dangerousness, produced serious doubts among some involved with the criminal justice system as to the value or the ethical propriety of taking such predictions seriously (American Psychiatric Association 1974). Mental health professionals have also lost confidence in their own predictive powers and now either make modest claims or concede that prediction of most harmful events is not within the realm of their expertise (American Psychological Association 1978).

Among attorneys, clinicians, and academicians who have carefully scrutinized the problem, little confidence is currently found in the capacity of any professional group to accurately predict violence. Nevertheless, such predictions must be made, and the mental health professional is still called upon to assist in the process. The prevailing view seems to be that prediction may, at times, rise to a level of accuracy that makes it worthy of consideration in making judgments within the civil and criminal justice systems. According to Monahan (1981), "there may be circumstances in which prediction is both empirically possible and ethically appropriate." This would appear to be especially true when predictions are limited to behavior likely to occur in a relatively short period of time.

While the proposition that mental health professionals cannot predict dangerousness is widely accepted, it must also be acknowledged that prediction is an everyday feature of other aspects of their clinical practice. This is especially true of medical practice, where the diagnostic process can be viewed as an effort to predict that the patient may experience certain incapacities. Diagnosis in medicine begins with an empirical approach in which a cluster of symptoms or behaviors is noted to have a predictable course. Individuals observed to have such a set of symptoms or signs are then labeled as having a particular type of disorder (Woodruff et al. 1974). Once the course of a disorder is known, various treatments can be used to determine if the course (or the prognosis) can be altered. This is the value of diagnosis as a predictive tool.

Without such prediction or prognostication, the efficacy of treatment could not be evaluated. Patients and relatives can then be advised as to what the outcome of a particular illness might be. Physicians can predict that individuals who demonstrate a particular cluster of symptoms will experience physical deterioration or perhaps social and occupational deterioration. Such physical or lifestyle predictions can be made with a high degree of probability. It is, of course, much more difficult for a physician to predict that the existence of a cluster of observable signs and symptoms will regularly be associated with future behavior, such as a violent act. Nevertheless, those accustomed to working within the medical model may readily find analogies between predicting that an individual with certain coronary artery deficiencies will develop heart failure if untreated, and predicting that an individual with certain psychological deficiencies will commit future crimes if untreated.

Mental Illness and Dangerousness

A prevailing assumption in both civil and criminal law indicates that the mentally ill are more dangerous than others. Society has traditionally viewed the mentally ill with distrust and fear. Its concern is greatest in dealing with mentally ill individuals who behave irrationally and who do not seem to respond to the social sanctions that control other citizens. Those who lack full capacity to respond to the punishments and reinforcements provided by the environment presumably are at high risk of harming themselves and others. Most of the time, we impose controls on the mentally ill because we fear that they may harm themselves. We are also concerned, however, that they may do harm to others.

Whether the mentally ill are actually more dangerous than others is unclear. A considerable amount of research has been done in this area, but all of the studies thus far are limited by problems of definition (Monahan and Steadman 1982). The degree to which we consider the mentally ill more or less dangerous than others depends in large part on how we define mental illness or mental disorder and by what criteria we define dangerousness. If those who have personality disorders or alcohol abuse problems are defined as mentally disordered, and if committing a crime is viewed as a manifestation of dangerousness, then we can say that substantial evidence exists that the mentally ill are highly dangerous. (We must be concerned with circularity in this type of thinking inasmuch as criminal conduct may be listed as one of the criteria for certain personality disorders, such as the antisocial personality disorder.) If, on the other hand, mental illness is defined as psychotic behavior, and committing a criminal act is considered a manifestation of dangerousness, some research indicates that the mentally ill are no more dangerous, and are sometimes less dangerous, than others—such as released prisoners (Steadman et al. 1978; Steadman 1981). This finding must also be qualified. It is possible that severely mentally ill individuals commit antisocial acts that would have led to criminal prosecution if society had not decided they were mentally ill. Conceivably, those who are seriously ill may commit more illegal acts than others, but those acts are not defined as crimes. We have no data to prove or disprove this possibility.

Dangerousness and Indeterminate Confinement

Society's natural response to the perception of dangerousness is self-protection. We seek to restrain those we perceive as dangerous so that they cannot hurt us. We may also try to rehabilitate them, either because we feel it is humane to do so or because we believe that rehabilitation provides more effective and less expensive protection than restraint. Suspected dangerous offenders are likely to be managed through a restraint/rehabilitation approach characterized by some form of indeterminate confinement. As a rule, indeterminate sentences are imposed primarily on persons who are considered highly dangerous, such as "psychopaths" or sex offenders. A few exceptions, however, do exist. Juveniles may be placed in partially indeterminate programs (i.e., up to age 18 or 21 years), where they are not viewed as dangerous but are felt to be in need of an extended period of supervision and treatment.

Partially indeterminate sentencing is also used for nondangerous offenders in jurisdictions that provide some limited range to the period of incarceration before parole. When parole is possible, however, a maximum sentence generally is specified, and the offender must almost always serve a minimum sentence. With the current popularity of presumptive sentencing, which requires judges to make relatively fixed sentences, even modified indeterminacy through parole is becoming less available (Forer 1980). The practice of offering "good time" (or guaranteed time off for good behavior) may help offenders gain freedom before their maximum term is expired, but its use cannot be directly related to the philosophy of indeterminate sentencing. Good behavior in prison may or may not be an indication that an offender can be safely released. The opportunity to offer time off for good behavior is primarily a means of providing authorities with a powerful reinforcement that helps them to retain control over prisoners.

Indeterminate sentencing in its purest form allows for indefinite restraints so that offenders can, in theory, be confined from one day to life. There are no maximum and no minimum sentences. Release is based simply on a belief that the probability offenders will engage in harmful behavior is low enough that concern with their welfare justifies setting them free. Should the level of suspected dangerousness remain high, and if society is unwilling to bear the risks of release, confinement could well be for life.

The restraint/rehabilitation model of indeterminate sentencing is similar to that used in the involuntary commitment of the mentally ill. It bears resemblance to the medical model insofar as it implies that some form of intervention will be utilized until the potentiality for undesirable behavior disappears. An important difference, however, is seen between the medical model as it is used in treating the mentally ill and how it is used in the restraint or rehabilitation of offenders. When society seeks to restrain or rehabilitate offenders, it is also likely to have some interest in punishing them. Mentally disordered offenders who are sentenced indeterminately are subject to more restraint than civil patients committed as mentally ill. They are rarely released as soon as they are judged to be nondangerous, nor are they regularly treated in the least restrictive manner consistent with public safety (Wexler 1976).

Currently, true indeterminate sentencing is rarely available to offenders. Only a few states have provisions for extending the period of detention of selected sex offenders to keep their maximum sentence indefinite (Dix 1983). In most programs, either statutory requirements or conservative practices can make early release (after a few weeks or months) rather unlikely. Problems of limited prison bed space and serious overcrowding, however, create pressures for releasing some inmates to make space available for others.

Critiques of Indeterminate Sentencing

The efficiency of an indeterminate program can be assessed in terms of the extent to which it continues to restrain the dangerous and releases the nondangerous as soon as possible. Another way of putting this is that it avoids false decisions—either a false negative decision that a truly dangerous person is not dangerous, or a false positive decision that a nondangerous person is dangerous (Monahan 1981). Efficiency is maximized when three conditions are met:

1. When clear criteria are present for identifying characteristics about individuals or their life situations that indicate a high potentiality for dangerousness. (Such characteristics would be readily apparent in a man who has a long history of child molestation, who admits to having powerful urges to have sex with children, and who is employed as a school teacher.)

2. When technologies are available to change the behavior of offenders or opportunities exist to change their environments in ways that will minimize the probability of subsequent dangerous behavior (for example, changing the motivations of child molesters or being able to place them in an environment with no children).

3. When reliable indicators show that potentially dangerous characteristics have been eliminated or substantially reduced. (In the absence of some gross alteration of the offender's physical condition, indicators of such behavioral change tend to be unreliable. As a rule, change must be inferred from the offender's behavior.)

These three conditions are difficult to fulfill. First of all, predictions of long-term dangerousness, which are of special importance in indeterminate sentencing programs, do not have a high degree of accuracy (Monahan 1981). The best predictor in this situation is a history of previously antisocial and violent behavior, but even this indicator is not always reliable (American Psychiatric Association 1974). Crimes such as exhibitionism, check forgery, or shoplifting, which have a high probability of being repeated, are generally not associated with a tendency to commit more violent crimes.

The second condition is also difficult to meet. The prevailing wisdom is that most technologies that modify characteristics of the individual offender, whether they be biological or psychological, are unlikely to be effective (MacNamara 1977). Unless the harmfulness of offenders is directed toward a specific target, such as small children, it is also difficult to create postrelease environments that diminish the likelihood of dangerous behavior. Undoubtedly, some postrelease interventions, such as job training, psychotherapy, or close supervision, make some difference in diminishing the probability of criminal behavior, but the degree of efficacy of any of these interventions is limited (Halleck and Witte 1977).

The most difficult problem, of course, is the absence of reliable indicators as to when an offender has made sufficient changes to be considered safe for release. As will be noted in a later section, conforming behavior of offenders in the institutional setting is not a reliable indicator that they are no longer dangerous. Nor can too much stock be put in statements by offenders that they no longer have the motivations or other characteristics that put them at risk of dangerous behavior. The most reliable indicators of change are aging or biological infirmity that serve to diminish the capacity of offenders to carry out the physical conduct involved in a harmful act. Sometimes, the passage of time may also create obvious and favorable changes in the environment to which offenders will be released. Offenders who molest only their own children, for example, may be better parole risks if they are released to their home after their children have grown up. Obviously, physical infirmity or the passage of time are not the most auspicious criteria on which to build an efficient indeterminate sentencing program.

Whether or not indeterminate programs are more or less efficient than determinate modes of sentencing, they are inefficient in certain obvious ways. Given current levels of knowledge and skill, such programs will always allow for the release of a certain number of individuals who will harm others and will allow restraint of some who are not dangerous. Those who demand greater public protection criticize indeterminate programs for releasing offenders too soon. Those concerned with the civil rights of offenders fear that offenders will be restrained unnecessarily.

Civil libertarians are especially concerned that, given the difficulty of prediction and the inadequacy of treatment methods, those who are responsible for managing indeterminate programs will resort to extraordinary methods of behavioral change. Indeterminately sentenced offenders may be particularly susceptible to becoming subjects of experimentation. Faced with so much uncertainty as to their future, they are often willing to try anything to gain freedom, even if this means accepting a remedy that may ultimately cause them serious harm and is repugnant to the sensibilities of society. In the past two decades, mentally disordered offenders have on many occasions been subjected to experiments that were potentially more harmful than helpful (Dix 1983). It is possible that indeterminate sentencing puts mentally disordered offenders at higher risk of such abuse.

Dangerousness and Fixed Sentencing

The existence of a mental disorder that is believed to be associated with a potentiality for dangerousness, in addition to triggering procedures that lead to a relatively indeterminate disposition, may also influence the court in determining the length of a fixed sentence. The possibility that the presence of a mental disorder might mitigate the harshness of punishment imposed during the sentencing phase of the criminal trial was briefly noted in the preceding chapter. Here, it must be noted that data relevant to the mental condition of offenders, particularly if that mental condition is believed to be associated with dangerousness, can also be utilized to justify a lengthier sentence. While offenders who are given fixed sentences are not usually classified as mentally disordered offenders to the extent that their disposition is directly related to their alleged mental illness and dangerousness, the role of mental health professionals in influencing their sentencing is an appropriate subject for this monograph.

Mental health clinicians have a long tradition of participating in the process of sentencing (Guttmacher 1958). In many jurisdictions, offenders are examined at psychiatric court clinics, where clinical reports are prepared and communicated directly to the judges who pass sentences. This informal reporting may never be subjected to cross-examination. In other jurisdictions, formal evaluations may be introduced to the court after the defendant has been convicted. These reports are available to both the defense and the prosecution, and the expert who prepared them is likely to be examined by both sides. Both formal and informal reporting may focus on the issue of dangerousness, but other factors related to the offender's mental state may be brought to the court's attention. The mitigating or aggravating quality of these factors is then considered in assessing the extent of the offender's penalty.

In those jurisdictions that give the judge some discretion in sentencing, evidence of mental disorders may have considerable influence on the length of sentence imposed. The mental health clinician who prepares a presentence evaluation for the court then becomes a key functionary in the sentencing process. Serious ethical problems arise when the mental health clinician is granted so much power to influence the sentencing process. These problems will be discussed in a later part of this chapter as well as in chapter 8.

Civil Rights of Offenders Committed to Specialized Programs

Because of all the potential transgressions on civil liberties of offenders that may result from diversion to specialized and indeterminate treatment programs, the courts have scrutinized these programs carefully. Some of the issues that have been litigated are relevant to all classes of mentally disordered offenders. They tend to assume the most prominence, however, in the context of indeterminate confinement. The major issues still in the process of being litigated will be briefly noted here.

1. *Is diversion to specialized treatment programs constitutional?* Efforts have been made to find specialized treatment programs unconstitutional under the equal protection and due process clauses of the 14th amendment. If little evidence exists that mentally disordered sex offenders constitute a special class of dangerous individuals who are actually treatable, then they may have been singled out for indeterminate confinement without a rational basis. Since they may be deprived of liberty for a longer period of time and under more restrictive circumstances than ordinary offenders, it can be argued that their specialized treatment violates their right to equal protection (LaFave and Scott 1972). The lack of precise definitions of dangerousness or mental impairment in most instances leading to specialized sentencing has also been viewed as violating the due process requirements of the Constitution (*Pearson v. Probate Court* 1940). It can be argued that current imprecise standards do not give an individual who is affected by the possibility of indeterminate commitment sufficient opportunity to know how to avoid this outcome. It is also possible that the lack of precision could encourage arbitrariness in the application of current standards by police, prosecutors, or the courts. Up until now, both equal protection and due process constitutional arguments have been rejected by higher courts.

2. *What procedural safeguards are available to offenders diverted to specialized treatment programs?* Recent Supreme Court decisions have tended to expand procedural safeguards for offenders who face specialized sentencing proceedings (*Specht v. Patterson* 1967; *Lockett v. Ohio* 1978). In such proceedings, defendants have the right to be present with counsel and the opportunity to be heard, to be confronted with and to cross-examine witnesses against them, and to offer evidence of their own. In related sentencing situations, where capital punishment is an option that can be imposed by the judge or jury, the Supreme Court has acknowledged an even greater need for care—so-called "super due process" (Radin 1980). At the very least, defendants in capital hearings are given full opportunity to present mitigating arguments and to attack arguments in support of aggravating considerations.

The question of whether offenders facing diversion to a specialized program can refuse to cooperate in the psychiatric examination to determine their need for treatment has not been clearly decided. It can be argued that cooperation in such an examination is equivalent to self-incrimination, and that under the fifth amendment offenders can refuse to be examined. With rare exceptions, the courts have not allowed this argument in cases involving diversion of sex offenders or other allegedly dangerous offenders (Dix 1983). Where the death penalty is involved, however, the Supreme Court appears to have given capital offenders the privilege of refusing to participate in examinations designed to determine if they are dangerous (*Estelle v. Smith* 1981).

Most states with specialized treatment programs have statutory provisions for release that require the participation of both the superintendent of the treatment institution and the committing court. The court can either reject the superintendent's recommendation or order conditional or unconditional release. In most programs, offenders are also provided with the right to periodic review of their status (Dix 1983).

3. *Do offenders sentenced to specialized treatment programs have a right to treatment?* If offenders are sentenced to indeterminate treatment programs and cannot be released until they have improved, it would appear that both their interest and society's interest would be best served if they received adequate treatment. The situation bears some resemblance to that of involuntarily committed mental patients who would also appear to be entitled to treatment. While lower courts have argued that such a right exists for civilly committed patients (*Donaldson v. O'Con-*

nor 1974), the Supreme Court has avoided ruling on this issue (*O'Connor v. Donaldson* 1975).

In some jurisdictions, mentally disordered offenders have been provided with a statutory right to treatment (*Rouse v. Cameron* 1966). The courts have also appeared to be especially interested in enforcing the right to treatment where mentally disordered offenders are sentenced to specialized treatment programs and housed in correctional institutions rather than security or public hospitals (*State v. Little* 1978). Right-to-treatment litigation also raises the question of adequacy of treatment for mentally disordered offenders. The courts have tended to rule that minimum standards of care are adequate (*in re Thompson* 1977).

Currently, the availability and adequacy of treatment varies from state to state. Treatment practices are partially controlled by court orders or statutes, but they are still heavily influenced by budgetary decisions, by legislative bodies, and by the security needs of the hospital. The clearest outcome of right-to-treatment litigation has been the influence on security hospitals to pay greater attention to treatment planning. Almost all security hospitals now formulate plans, which are recorded in the patient's chart (Kerr and Roth in press). Most hospitals also hold regular staff conferences in which the offender's progress is assessed. Whether such an administrative focus on treatment actually results in the provision of better treatment is uncertain. Improved record keeping and conferences may do little more than increase the likelihood that patients will not be ignored. The adequacy of treatment will still be determined by the availability of funds and skilled professionals.

4. *Do specially sentenced defenders have a right to refuse treatment?* The extent to which ordinary mental patients or any group of mentally disordered offenders have a right to refuse treatment is still undetermined. Both groups, however, have been substantially protected from certain types of unwanted treatment by the courts. Many court rulings have involved cases of mentally ill offenders who are viewed as having a high risk of being subjected to experimental procedures or coerced into "volunteering" for them. Currently, interventions are regulated primarily on the basis of their alleged intrusiveness. Behavior modification, based on aversive conditioning or on removing privileges and then replacing them contingent on good behavior, is strictly monitored by the courts and will have a high likelihood of being terminated (*Mackey v. Procunier* 1973; *Clonce v. Richardson* 1974). This seems to hold whether participation in such programs is voluntary or

forced. Electroconvulsive treatment remains so controversial, and its use is so burdened by legal restrictions, that it is almost never imposed on mentally disordered offenders. Experimental psycho-surgery has been prohibited even when offenders volunteer for it (*Kaimowitz v. Department of Mental Health* 1973).

The major controversy these days revolves around whether civ-illy committed mental patients and formally designated mentally disordered offenders have a right to refuse psychotropic medica-tion. Recent litigation in Massachusetts and New Jersey has ex-panded the right of refusal of civilly committed patients who ap-pear to be competent and present no immediate threat to their own safety or that of others (*Rennie v. Klein* 1978; *Rogers v. Okin* 1980). While the major cases have not yet been litigated to the ex-tent that they provide clear guidelines, mental health professionals have learned to be cautious in forcing medication on patients in any setting. Whether this has significantly curtailed the use of psychotropic drugs with involuntary mental patients or mentally disordered offenders is unclear. Patients can still be treated in-voluntarily if adjudicated incompetent or in emergency situations where they are a threat to themselves or others. Even patients whose incompetence and dangerousness have not been proven can, in most jurisdictions, still be treated against their will. A common practice these days, which meets with the approval of at least one of the courts dealing with this litigation, is to have a consultant examine patients who are felt to need treatment but who are re-fusing it. If the consultant recommends treatment, it is given.

Relationship of the Concept of "Dangerousness" to the Stability of the Criminal Justice System

In the previous two chapters, it was noted that incompetent and insane offenders can be viewed by the criminal justice system as exceptions who prove the rule that all other offenders are com-petent or sane. Does the criminal justice system also view danger-ous offenders who are sentenced with varying degrees of indeter-minacy as exceptions to the rule that fixed sentences serve the purposes of criminal justice? The answer in this instance is some-what equivocal. On the one hand, the criminal justice system does limit the number of offenders it treats in specialized programs, just as it limits the number of incompetent and insane offenders. The potential dangerousness of the majority of offenders is never formally considered. In this sense, mentally disordered sex of-fenders and others sentenced indeterminately are exceptional. On the other hand, mentally disordered sex offenders are only partially diverted from ordinary criminal justice practices. Whether they are housed in prisons or in maximum security hospitals, they are treated more like prisoners than like mental patients. Unlike the incompetent or the insane, they may be viewed as patients during only one small part of the day or week, while the rest of the time they are viewed as ordinary prisoners.

I have previously argued that limiting diversion and taking an all-or-none approach to questions of incompetency and insanity serves to preserve the integrity of a system that emphasizes retributive justice. The same arguments are, in part, relevant to the issue of dangerousness. If the criminal justice system dealt with too many offenders through specialized sentencing and treatment programs, it would gradually move toward a restraint/rehabilitation model in which its response to crime would be influenced by the characteristics of the offender rather than by the nature of the crime. Limiting the extent of specialized disposition appears to add stability to a retributive system.

Clinical Issues

The Power of Predicting Dangerousness

As a clinician who has worked in forensic settings and has participated in civil commitment proceedings, I have always been impressed with how seriously and respectfully the public and courts deal with psychiatric predictions of dangerousness. (The previously noted skepticism of some attorneys and academicians is not characteristic of others who work in the criminal justice system.) Other clinicians with similar experiences have also noted that the predictions of experts tend to exert a powerful influence on judicial decisions (Robitscher 1980). This contrasts somewhat with the tendency of the public and sometimes of the courts to view expert testimony on issues such as competency or insanity as being arbitrary and unscientific.

It is possible that the acceptance expert testimony receives in this instance is not determined by public trust in the predictive capacities of experts but is, in large part, related to the possible outcomes their testimony supports. If the expert's prediction of dangerousness is ignored, and the offender commits a violent act, the court has made a harmful mistake. No such risk is taken if diagnoses of incompetency or insanity are ignored. In the latter instance, only the offender may suffer and no direct threat is made to public safety. Particularly during periods when concern for public protection outweighs civil liberty interests, predictions of dangerousness that call for specialized or increased restraint are likely to be taken more seriously by the courts, regardless of their reliability. At the same time, predictions that an individual is not dangerous tend to be given much closer scrutiny.

Mental health professionals who testify in court should be aware that the court's perception of their skills is not always accurate. Particularly in dealing with the issue of dangerousness, experts can wield a degree of influence that may not be justified by their knowledge or demonstrated expertise. Mental health professionals should learn to use their power to influence judges and juries wisely and acknowledge the limits of their expertise when presenting their testimony. Monahan (1981) proposes that clinicians consider 14 questions in attempting to predict violent behavior.

1. Is it a prediction of violent behavior that is being requested?
2. Am I professionally competent to offer an estimate of the probability of future violence?
3. Are any issues of personal or professional ethics involved in this case?
4. Given my answers to the above questions, is this case an appropriate one in which to offer a prediction?
5. What events precipitated the question of the person's potential for violence, and in what context did these events take place?
6. What are the person's relevant demographic characteristics?
7. What is the person's history of violent behavior?
8. What is the base rate of violent behavior among individuals of this person's background?
9. What are sources of stress in the person's current environment?
10. What cognitive and affective factors indicate that the person may be predisposed to cope with stress in a violent manner?
11. What cognitive and affective factors indicate that the person may be predisposed to cope with stress in a nonviolent manner?
12. How similar are the contexts in which the person has used violent coping mechanisms in the past to those in which the person likely will function in the future?
13. In particular, who are the likely victims of the person's violent behavior, and how available are they?
14. What means does the person possess to commit violence?

These questions require the evaluator to take an interactional approach and to be constantly aware that violent behavior cannot be conceptualized in terms of the individual alone; it must also be understood in terms of the environments in which a susceptible individual is likely to interact. The approach here is relativistic and requires that dangerousness be viewed in probabilistic terms.

Monahan (1981) also provides guidelines for reporting evaluations of dangerousness (violence). He urges clinicians to restrict their reports to statements of the probability of a violent act's occurring in a particular environment over a defined period of time. He further advises clinicians that, when possible, they should avoid conclusory statements that an individual is dangerous and should leave the ultimate adjudication of dangerousness to the court. This approach provides the court, or whatever agency is determining the issue of dangerousness, with as much expert information as the clinician can legitimately provide. The determination of the degree of potential harmfulness that requires some type of intervention, such as increased or continued restraint, is then left to those who represent the community's interest.

Clinical Problems in Evaluating Dangerousness

The criminal justice system calls for clinical evaluation of dangerousness, and therefore clinical prediction of dangerousness, in four types of situations:

1. When decisions must be made whether individuals found incompetent to stand trial or not guilty by reason of insanity should be released or restrained in a hospital through some process of commitment.
2. When incarcerated offenders are felt to be mentally ill and it is feared that their mental illness will be associated with violent behavior.
3. When defendants are evaluated for sentencing.
4. When institutionalized offenders are evaluated for release from indeterminate sentencing programs.

The first and fourth categories deal primarily with decisions to release or retain offenders. The second and third deal with decisions to place offenders in programs where they may be treated differently than ordinary offenders or with decisions as to the degree of punishment. Each of these evaluations poses somewhat different clinical problems. Problems involved in decisions to release insanity acquittees have already been discussed and will not be reviewed here.

1. *Predicting the dangerousness of those found incompetent to stand trial.* Individuals who have been found incompetent to stand trial and who do not make substantial progress toward recovery must eventually be committed under the ordinary rules of civil commitment or be discharged. The continued civil commitment of incompetent offenders must be justified by evidence of their dangerousness to themselves or others. Periodic review of the mental illness and dangerousness of these offenders is required.

The task of the evaluator in this situation is to assess the dangerousness of individuals who have not technically been convicted of a crime but have involuntarily been institutionalized. One problem with doing this has already been noted in chapter 3. If the only evidence of dangerousness is proof that offenders have committed the crimes with which they are charged, such proof may not be available. Other problems of evaluation are created when these individuals have been restrained in an institutional environment for a long period of time. The amount of time that may have elapsed between their having been accused of committing a crime and the request for psychiatric assessment of dangerousness may vary from a few months to years. During this time, they have been living in environments quite different from those in which their crimes were likely to have been committed, and little current data are available as to their likely response to environmental situations previously associated with their criminal behavior. Available information as to their most recent behavior in the institution may not help to predict dangerousness, since such behavior does not usually parallel behavior in the free world. Some people will be difficult management problems and perhaps even violent within institutions but might be much more compliant in a free environment. More commonly, offenders behave in a socially acceptable manner as long as they are in a structured setting, such as a prison or hospital. Once this structure disappears, their propensity for violence may increase.

It is also likely that at the time of evaluation persons found incompetent to stand trial will have been treated with neuroleptic medication. This may significantly alter their conduct in the institution where they have been retained, as well as their conduct during the course of their evaluation. There will be a decreased likelihood of their indulging in antisocial conduct as long as they continue to take antipsychotic or neuroleptic drugs. Because of their medicated state, they may appear calm and rational during the evaluation. There is usually no way, however, of knowing how they would behave without their medication or whether they would continue to take it.

Another problem is that the particular mental disorder that determines incompetency may have little to do with the propensity of offenders to commit violent acts in the future. Many offenders who are found incompetent to stand trial have disorders that develop subsequent to their crimes. These disorders may be unrelated to other mental characteristics (such as the presence of personality disorders) that may be associated with a high probability of their subsequently committing crimes. The improvement of the condition that led to the initial finding of incompetency does not negate the possibility of future dangerousness.

2. *Predicting dangerousness in the prison setting.* The problems involved in deciding when offenders imprisoned under the ordinary criminal code are at risk for violence related to a mental illness are not as formidable as those encountered in most evaluations of dangerousness. These persons are sent for evaluation after they have already been violent or have been acting strangely. The clinician has some evidence of recent behavior that may be a predictor of future violence. The clinician is also being asked to predict the occurrence of violence in one particular environment, the prison, and behavior that puts offenders at risk of being violent in that environment is relatively easy to define.

Prisons are characterized by a great deal of violence. Offenders can avoid violence only by being extremely mindful of all the stimuli in their environment. Any impairment in reality testing increases the risks of their being involved in violent acts. Individuals who make threats based on delusional perceptions of their environment, for example, are likely to invite a violent response. Generally, those with impaired capacities to evaluate the risks and benefits of a violent act are at high risk, because few nonviolent alternative behaviors are available to them, and because violence in prison may actually be condoned by the prevailing subculture. A prediction of violence may have considerable short-term utilitarian value in the prison setting, since the environment can be made more benign or substantially changed by transferring the disturbed inmate to a hospital unit.

3. *Predicting dangerousness for sentencing purposes.* In a variety of instances, presentence clinical assessments of dangerousness are

requested by the criminal justice system to determine how a defendant's potential for violence will influence the sentencing decision. If the assessment predicts a high likelihood of future violence, the offender is likely to be sent to an institution where concern with security is high and privileges are few. As a rule, however, clinical predictions of dangerousness for sentencing purposes are primarily used to determine the length of a fixed sentence, whether capital punishment is to be imposed, or whether the offender will be sent to a specialized treatment program. In all of these evaluations, the clinician is concerned with helping to make dispositions that impose varying degrees and durations of restraint upon offenders.

The clinical task of predicting dangerousness for sentencing purposes is a much more difficult exercise than the more familiar task of predicting dangerousness for purposes of civil commitment. This is because the consequences of prediction are more likely to be harmful to offenders. They will usually appreciate that the examining clinician has enormous power to influence their destiny. They know that, to the extent they can persuade the clinician that they are nondangerous, they will receive a more favorable disposition. Obviously, such a situation does not encourage offenders to be spontaneous or honest. Unless they are ignorant or misled as to the purpose of the examination, they will emphasize their psychological strengths and minimize their weaknesses. They are also likely to view the mental health professional as an adversary, as someone to persuade or to "con" into writing a favorable report.

Faced with a resistant or deceptive subject, the clinician must overcome major handicaps in order to conduct an adequate examination. The evaluation of patients in general proceeds most efficiently when their honest self-disclosure is maximized. Clinical evaluation is most likely to be reliable when patients present adequate histories, respond in as spontaneous a manner as possible to the examiner's questions, and try to recall events and feelings they may not have been aware of at the beginning of the interview. When such responses are not forthcoming, the clinician must either develop special techniques for evaluating resistant clients or must find a way of making clients less resistant.

Elsewhere, I have described a variety of techniques for evaluating reluctant subjects (Halleck 1967). These center on evaluating the interactional process between the examiner and the offender, rather than on the actual content of the offender's statements. Emphasis is placed on the manner in which the offender deals with a variety of challenges, such as questioning his or her truthfulness, or how the offender responds to diversionary techniques, such as general discussions of religion or philosophy. The extent of information revealed by such techniques is limited, but it may be sufficient to influence the clinician's opinion as to the offender's dangerousness. Serious ethical problems accompany this approach, of course. The examiner is using clinical techniques that are less than straightforward in order to obtain information that might be used to deprive the offender of liberty.

The alternative of making the client less resistant is unlikely to be accomplished without some deception. Sometimes, the clinician is able to exploit the trust that most people have in mental health professionals and to deceive clients into believing that the expert is acting only in their best interest. This can be done by simply not explaining the nature of the interview to offenders or by giving a less-than-candid response to inquiries concerning its purpose. The ethical problems here are formidable and will be discussed in greater detail in the chapter on ethics.

In the absence of extraordinary skill or blatant disregard for ethical considerations, evaluation of dangerousness in the sentencing situation is not likely to be very accurate. Conceivably, many evaluators are "conned" into perceiving offenders as more peaceable than they actually are. More cynical or "hardened" evaluators come to pride themselves on their ability to avoid being "conned." They are at risk of finding deceptiveness and, therefore, dangerousness among those who may actually be truthful and non-dangerous. Clinicians, of course, should learn to be extremely humble with regard to their predictions of dangerousness in this kind of situation. Their skills are meager, and their potential for doing harm is great.

4. *Assessment of dangerousness at the time of release.* Assessment of the dangerousness of convicted offenders who are being considered for release may be required when the offender has not been given a fixed sentence and when release is determined by some type of parole or review board. In jurisdictions that have indeterminate sentencing, periodic evaluation of the offender's progress is required by statute. In addition to being concerned with the offender's behavior within the institution, parole and review boards also wish to know whether the offender has made significant psychological changes. The task of the expert in this situation is similar but not identical to that involved in discharging civilly committed patients, including incompetent offenders and insanity acquittees who have been committed on the basis of

dangerousness. (Two important differences are that offenders who are sentenced indeterminately have been convicted of a crime and are likely to have been diagnosed as having personality disorders rather than psychotic diagnoses.)

When consideration of dangerousness is a factor in determining release of mentally disordered offenders, an earlier determination has usually been made that the person is dangerous. If the offender is to be released, a prediction of nondangerousness must be made. In this situation, the prediction of nondangerousness is something more than just a nonprediction of dangerousness. The predictor must negate a previous prediction made by a mental health professional, which the courts may have taken seriously enough to justify the imposition of a specialized form of sentencing. To predict nondangerousness, the evaluator must be able to argue that the probabilities that certain offenders will commit dangerous acts have substantially changed and are now so low that society should be willing to tolerate whatever limited risks are entailed by releasing them.

The problem of assessing a shift from dangerousness to non-dangerousness is particularly difficult when the mental disorder on which the original assessment was based is a personality or sexual dysfunction disorder. These disorders may have been, in part, diagnosed on the basis of the illegal act itself (Monahan and Davis 1983). If this is the case, little opportunity exists to look for changes in symptoms as an index of improvement, since the major symptoms of diagnostic importance are criminal acts that may be difficult to perform in prison. If the personality disorder is characterized by behavior other than, or in addition to, the criminal act, it will still be difficult to determine how much these non-criminal characteristics will have changed. Symptoms such as alcohol or substance abuse, which are often associated with the diagnosis of a personality disorder, cannot be observed in an institutional setting where such drugs are usually not available. If offenders who have committed sex crimes only when intoxicated are imprisoned for months or years, and then claim that they should be released because they have stopped drinking and do not intend to drink when they are released, there is no way to confirm the reliability of their assertions. Still another problem is that offenders who are evaluated for release will, much like those who are being sentenced, try to conceal as many of their deviant tendencies as possible. Some who have personality disorders are likely to be quite skilled in presenting themselves in the best possible light.

The difficulty of predicting the nondangerousness of indeterminately sentenced offenders may be slightly attenuated by the context in which the evaluation is done. This is one prediction that can, at least, be done at a leisurely pace. The offender is usually institutionalized and can be examined more than once. The data on which the original prediction of violence was based should be available. Considerable time will have elapsed between the initial prediction and the later evaluation, and even though offenders have spent that time in the artificial environment of a custodial institution, it is possible to make some assessments as to how their situation has changed. Factors such as aging, intercurrent illness, religious conversion, relief of emotional problems, learning new skills, or changes in the environment to which the offender will be released may diminish the probability of future dangerousness and can be cited as evidence of nondangerousness.

Emerging Legal Issues

While specialized programs for sex offenders or other abnormal offenders may be disappearing, it may also be premature to sound the death knell for the restraint/rehabilitation model under which they are diverted. The development of new technologies of treatment and a variety of social considerations, which I will elaborate in the final chapter, may change this situation in the near future. It is useful to note here, however, that the civil libertarian attacks on indeterminate sentencing programs have been somewhat muted in the past few years. There appears to be no major constitutional challenge to the legitimacy of specialized treatment programs on the horizon. Nor have any new issues been raised in the past several years that would substantially influence the procedural rights of diverted offenders, their right to treatment, or their right to refuse treatment.

The Future Role of Mental Health Experts in the Sentencing Process

Perhaps the most interesting litigation in the near future will involve the participation of mental health professionals in the sentencing process. It is difficult to predict whether differential sentencing of offenders, based on how mental disorders influence either dangerousness or liability, will increase or decrease in the future. Recent legal trends can be cited to predict change in either direction. Current antagonism toward indeterminate sentencing and parole and the new enthusiasm for determinate sentencing, which gives less discretion to the judge, are trends that would appear to be decreasing the consideration of mental disorder in the sentencing process. Some trends, however, augur for changes in the other direction. These include the following:

1. *A revived interest in restricting the number of insanity acquittals while allowing information concerning the defendant's emotional disturbance to influence the degree of the fixed penalty imposed at the time of sentencing.* At first glance, proposals to emphasize psychological factors at the sentencing rather than at the guilt determination phase of the trial bear some similarity to ideas advanced many years ago by such rehabilitationists as Lady Barbara Wootton (1968) and Dr. Karl Menninger (1959). These reformers were concerned less, however, with how much punishment should be imposed upon offenders than with the extent of necessary restraints while efforts were made to rehabilitate them. Current interest in considering the mental condition of offenders at the time of sentencing tends to be based on a "deserts" model of justice. It is assumed that the concept of deserts sets the upper and lower limits of punishment, and that the presence of mental illness can then be considered in "fine tuning" the exact degree of punishment (Morris 1982).

2. In addition to greater emphasis on determinate sentencing, *a new emphasis on presumptive sentencing in which the judge, whether restricted to upper and lower penalties, must also consider both mitigating and aggravating circumstances in determining the length of sentence* (Frankel 1972). Evidence of mental illness at the time of the crime is generally considered to be a mitigating circumstance. Evidence that a defendant poses a high risk of serious future criminal activity because of a mental disorder associated with dangerousness may be a basis for imposing a sentence longer than a presumptively proper one. It is possible, but by no means certain, that states that accept a presumptive sentencing doctrine will become increasingly concerned with relating mental disorder to sentencing.

3. *The increasing use of mental health professionals to consider the issue of mental disorder in determining whether those convicted of murder in the first degree shall receive life imprisonment or be executed.* In a series of decisions culminating in the 1978 case of *Lockett v. Ohio*, the United States Supreme Court ruled that, in accord with the eighth amendment, the sentence of death can be imposed only after a sentencing hearing in which the prosecution

and defense are permitted to introduce evidence related to a wide variety of potentially aggravating and mitigating considerations (*Lockett v. Ohio* 1978). This constitutionally mandated individualization of the sentencing process has already resulted in the use of mental health testimony to explore the influence of mental disorder on the imposition of the ultimate penalty.

Assuming that the reports mental health clinicians provide to courts will have increased importance in determining sentencing, the criminal justice system will have to carefully scrutinize current practices regarding informal reporting. In jurisdictions where informal reporting is common, reports of mental health experts that influence sentencing are not likely to be available to the defendant. Experts may simply send brief notes to judges or might even have informal conversations with them, at which time sentencing recommendations are presented. Thus the defendant is deprived of the opportunity to contest the accuracy of the expert's findings in an adversarial process. In effect, the defendant's fate may be dependent upon the wisdom and judgment of a party who never appears in the courtroom.

It is hoped that informal reporting will become less common in the future. Mental health professionals and judges are increasingly aware of the potential hazards of the practice. The Supreme Court has also mandated the necessity of exposing the testimony of mental health professionals to an adversarial process when indeterminate sentencing to a sex crime program or capital punishment is at issue (*Gardner v. Florida* 1977).

Even when psychiatric reporting is formalized, however, problems may arise when information is obtained and reported under circumstances in which the offender's rights are not protected. This has been a special problem in death penalty cases. In one case, information gained in an examination designed to determine an offender's competency to stand trial was later used at the capital sentencing phase of the trial as evidence of that offender's dangerousness (*Estelle v. Smith* 1981). While the Supreme Court declared this practice to be a violation of the offender's fifth and sixth amendment rights, the case has nevertheless alerted many mental health professionals and attorneys to the problems that can arise when psychiatric involvement in sentencing is not subject to strict rules of legal procedure.

The new interest in using mental health professionals to testify as to mitigating or aggravating circumstances at the sentencing phase raises many interesting questions, primarily because few consistent standards have been set to guide either the expert or the court in determining what factors are aggravating or mitigating. Is being intoxicated a mitigating factor? Being mentally retarded? Will jurisdictions eventually have to develop standards, similar to those of the American Law Institute for determining insanity, in order to help the judge or jury decide how much disability is actually mitigating? (Some states, such as North Carolina, have already done so.)

Questions raised by expert testimony that a mental disorder is an aggravating factor are even more troubling. For example, how should dangerousness be defined for purposes of sentencing? What degree of dangerousness must be determined to consider its presence as an aggravating factor? How should experts be allowed to testify as to dangerousness? The last question is especially interesting. Conclusory testimony as to an offender's dangerousness has become common in death penalty hearings in some jurisdictions. Psychiatrists have testified conclusively and emphatically that individuals facing the death penalty were extremely dangerous, while making no effort to document or even to discuss the basis of their predictions. Such testimony is difficult to rebut, unless experts are also available to defendants and will testify that they are not dangerous. Where experts for the defense are not available, conclusory testimony by prosecution-employed psychiatrists can be instrumental in rulings favoring the death penalty.

The use of expert testimony in the sentencing process has thus far received much less scrutiny than similar uses of testimony in pretrial incompetency hearings or insanity trials. This situation is unlikely to remain static. It is reasonable to predict that, as awareness of problems associated with such testimony grows, we will see an increasing formalization of the procedures under which offenders are examined for sentencing and under which experts present their opinions to the courts.

CHAPTER 6

Mental Disorder Resulting in Transfer
from Prison to Security Hospital

A CERTAIN NUMBER of convicted offenders exhibit symptoms of a mental disorder while in prison. Some members of this group may have been mentally disturbed long before their incarceration. Their symptoms may have gone undetected as they progressed through the legal process, or their original disorder may not have been viewed as severe enough to warrant a response, such as diversion, until their symptoms were exacerbated in the course of imprisonment. Other offenders who develop mental disorders in prison may have been free of symptoms prior to their arrest. In many cases, their symptoms could be viewed as a response to the stresses of incarceration.

Identification and Disposition of
Prison-to-Hospital Transfers

Identification

Obviously, not all prisoners who suffer from mental disorders are formally labeled as mentally disordered offenders. Only those whose disorders are especially blatant, or especially troubling to the prison, are likely to be transferred to a separate treatment-oriented facility. Such transfers are authorized by statutes that temporarily divert the prisoner into a new caretaking system. When transfer requires a legal process, such as filing a petition or affidavit (with or without a judicial hearing), the prisoner is formally identified as a mentally disordered offender.

In a study of institutionalized mentally disordered offenders in 1978, 51 percent of those admitted to maximum security hospitals during that year were transferred from correctional settings (Monahan et al. 1983). Transferred offenders do not usually retain their diverted status very long and are returned to prison when their condition improves. Since their average length of stay is about 6 months, they represent a smaller percentage of permanent residents than of admissions to security hospitals. In the study cited, these cases made up 36 percent of the institutionalized mentally disordered offender population.

In all classes of mentally disordered offenders discussed in previous chapters, diversion is based on criteria that have been formulated into legal standards. A judicial agency relies on relatively explicit standards to determine an offender's competency, insanity, or sexual dangerousness. In the case of transferred offenders, the standards for diversion are somewhat less clearly defined. Some states, such as Iowa and Wisconsin, initiate a process of formal civil commitment when transferring prisoners to security hospitals. In such cases, the standards for transfer are the same as the standards for civil commitment. But in other jurisdictions, the only formal criterion for transfer, especially when the prisoner does not contest the move, is the diagnosis of a serious mental disorder. This may be true even when the jurisdiction adheres to a recent ruling of the Supreme Court and requires that the transfer be preceded by substantial procedural protection (*Vitek v. Jones* 1980).

Initiation of Transfers

Decisions to transfer mentally disordered prisoners to hospitals are initiated by prison psychiatrists or psychologists but must be approved by prison administrators. Certain practical considerations are involved in making the decision to transfer. Jail or prison authorities must be aware of the offender's symptoms, must define them as manifestations of a mental disorder, and must decide that offenders who are transferred cannot be managed in an ordinary correctional setting. The realities of prison life are such that these considerations may lead to the transfer of some who might not be considered mentally disordered in the free world, as well as a failure to transfer others who would.

Decisions to transfer are, in large part, based on the nature of symptoms and how they are manifested. Certain symptoms of mental disorder are likely to be unnoticed in prison. Prisoners may cry, become mute, hallucinate, experience serious inability to think clearly, lose weight, fail to sleep for long periods of time, and be plagued with overpowering anxiety without anyone's noticing their plight. Should they complain, their symptomatology may simply be viewed as a normal response to incarceration. If they complain too consistently, they may be viewed as "manipulators" or "troublemakers." In any environment in which complaining about symptoms of emotional disorder can have more unpleasant than rewarding consequences, people tend to express their suffering by complaining about physical or somatic symptoms. Prisoners often develop serious psychosomatic or psychophysiologic complaints, which become a "ticket" for seeking help. The official medical response to such complaints in jails and prisons is likely to be reassurance and prescription of palliative medication. Little or no effort may be made to identify a mental disorder, and transfer may not even be considered.

The response of prison officials is quite different when complaints or behavioral variations are accompanied by self-destructive acts. Any type of self-destructive act that is noticed by officials, including self-mutilation, ingestion of a drug overdose, or attempt at hanging, will lead to the person's being defined as mentally disordered. Transfer is then likely. As a rule, prison officials will respond only to overt and serious suicidal attempts, not threats. Offenders who threaten suicide may temporarily be put under restrictions to reduce the likelihood of their harming themselves. But until they actually hurt themselves, they may simply be considered manipulative.

Inmates are also likely to be labeled as mentally disordered if their symptoms are associated with violence or the threat of violence. It is never entirely clear, however, why some violent inmates are labeled mentally disordered and others are not. The threat or performance of a violent act in the prison setting does not automatically trigger a suspicion of mental illness. Prison offers many reasons to be violent, most of which are viewed as rational by both inmates and administrators. These include fights over territory or contraband, rape, and defense against rape. Assault or threat of assault is so common in prison that it is usually viewed as normal behavior, subject only to disciplinary control and not needing any special form of treatment. Even assaults against custodial personnel are not necessarily viewed as signs of a mental disorder. In segregated disciplinary units, such behavior as cursing or hurling excrement at custodial personnel may be viewed as evidence of recalcitrance or "psychopathy" (Toch 1977).

A violent act is most likely to elicit psychiatric examination and possible transfer when it is viewed as irrational by prison administrators or when its perpetrator is viewed as deviant or "strange." Inmates who appear to be withdrawn and who attack other inmates in full view of custodial officers are likely candidates for transfer. So are inmates who express bizarre motivations to explain their assaultiveness. Another group of violent offenders likely to be considered mentally disordered includes inmates who impress correctional administrators as being unresponsive to the threat of disciplinary sanctions, such as being kept for longer periods of time in punitive segregation. Those who continue to misbehave in segregation units and who appear willing to stay there indefinitely may eventually be viewed as desirable candidates for transfer.

Prison administrators also appear to be diligent in transferring inmates who are viewed as possible targets of violence as a result of having a mental disorder. Mentally ill prisoners are in some jeopardy of being exploited by predatory inmates. They may also be viewed as irritants by others. Offenders who are obviously mentally disturbed and who show poor judgment in relating to aggressive inmates are likely to be transferred quickly, or they will be moved to protective custody units.

Inmates and civil libertarian attorneys show some concern that assertive inmates who "stir up" other inmates or verbally challenge correctional procedures are in jeopardy of being labeled mentally disordered and "shipped off" to a hospital. This is an understandably tempting option for prison administrators, which is most likely to be exercised when transfers are not reviewed by the courts. In some instances, prison authorities may feel they must resort to such practices to sustain a certain degree of institutional stability or to prevent riots. These days, however, the use of transfer to "cool" dissent does not occur frequently. Prison administrators have been sensitized to this misuse of the transfer process and are restrained from abusing it, both by their greater self-consciousness and by the possibility of judicial review.

Other Factors Influencing Transfer

Two facilities are always involved in the transfer process, and the operational needs of each institution will have some influence on who is eventually transferred. Even with the new procedural restraints imposed upon correctional institutions, they can still attempt to increase the number of inmates transferred by encouraging mental health professionals to emphasize the severity of their disturbance. An institution's assessment of the severity of an offender's mental disorder will, in part, be influenced by its current degree of stability and its resources. In an overcrowded prison with considerable recent violence, prison administrators and mental health professionals will understandably feel pressure to transfer marginally disturbed offenders. If, on the other hand, the institution is in a quiescent period, and if it has at least adequate treatment facilities, it will not be eager to seek transfer.

The response of the security hospital toward transfer will also limit the number of inmates who are transferred. Although most security hospitals are required by statute to accept all persons who are transferred, they also have the power to return such inmates whenever they decide their health is restored. Also, overcrowding may prompt security hospital staff to return inmates to prison quickly when they do not appear to be treatable or are seen as security risks. Prison authorities soon learn that little is gained by transferring inmates under these circumstances.

This situation includes some risk that troubling or troublesome inmates may be shuttled back and forth between institutions without receiving adequate treatment. To avoid this possibility, most prison and hospital authorities try to reach some kind of agreement as to which types of prisoners are most suitable for transfer and what length of time they are likely to be treated. As a rule, security hospitals tend to be gracious in accepting and treating transferred prisoners, as long as the correctional institution does not flood the hospital with "troublemakers." Likewise, the prison is often gracious in accepting returned offenders, as long as prison authorities believe the hospital has made a reasonable effort to treat them.

Reasons for Seeking or Avoiding Transfer

There are obvious reasons why inmates might welcome transfer and less obvious reasons why they might not. Transferred inmates are more likely to receive needed treatment in the hospital than in the prison setting. The transfer may also allow them to temporarily escape an intolerable situation in which they fear violent assault by other prisoners or disciplinary action by correctional officials. It is also true that custodial regulations in security hospitals are usually less stringent than those in prison and that hospital inmates are likely to receive more privileges. Given these considerations, it would appear that most offenders who perceive themselves as needing help would not resist transfer. Nevertheless, many inmates, including some who are greatly in need of treatment, do resist it for reasons they perceive as compelling.

Offenders can, in the long run, be harmed as a result of transfer. Until fairly recently, convicted prisoners who were transferred to a maximum-security hospital risked automatic civil commitment to the same institution even after their sentence had expired (*Baxstrom v. Herold* 1966). This situation has been partially remedied by the Supreme Court, insofar as commitment following expiration of sentence is no longer automatic, but offenders transferred to security hospitals are still at risk of being committed through new civil procedures after their sentence has expired. Offenders transferred to security hospitals may also be compromised in their capacity to obtain parole. Members of parole boards may reason that individuals who cannot adjust to a correctional institution probably cannot adjust in society. They may also fear that offenders who are mentally disordered may be exceptionally dangerous. Even if parole is not a consideration, transferred inmates may lose "good time," or time off for good behavior. Inmates who are transferred must also deal with the stigma of being labeled mentally ill. Throughout our society, and certainly in the correctional setting, considerable loss of prestige attaches to being labeled "mad" rather than "bad" (Halleck 1967). Finally, inmates may fear that, if they become mental patients, they will lose the right to resist unwanted and intrusive treatment, such as drug therapy or behavior modification (Churgin 1983).

Ultimately, offenders are most likely to benefit from transfer when they are provided effective treatment in security hospitals in as brief a period as possible and then returned immediately to the prison. Data indicating that transferred inmates are kept in security hospitals for an average of only 6 months suggest that this is the usual outcome (Monahan et al. 1983). In some instances, however, inmates have been confined to hospitals for much longer periods of time and have not been treated effectively. This has engendered fear among many inmates as to the consequences of unmonitored transfer and has led to litigation designed to protect their rights in the transfer process.

Procedural Protections of Transferred Prisoners

The earliest litigation designed to protect the rights of transferred prison inmates was based on the argument that offenders transferred to mental hospitals were entitled to the same legal protection as other persons committed to a mental hospital. In 1966, the Supreme Court used this equal protection argument to rule that inmates committed to a mental hospital after their original sentence had expired had to be committed under existing civil commitment standards or be released (*Baxstrom v. Herold* 1966). The Court did not apply this same reasoning to inmates who were to be transferred while still serving their sentences. Two lower federal courts, however, did accept this argument (*Schuster v. Herold* 1969; *Matthews v. Hardy* 1969).

In 1980, the Supreme Court expanded the procedural protection of inmates recommended for transfer while still serving a sentence. It did not, however, invoke an equal protection analysis. At the time, the civil commitment statute of Nebraska, the state involved in the litigation, had been declared unconstitutional, so that the equal protection comparison was not possible. The Court instead focused on the due process rights of transferred prisoners and reasoned that offenders had a protected liberty interest in not being transferred. The Court noted that these persons were entitled to the following procedural protections:

1. Written notice to the prisoner that a transfer to a mental hospital is being considered.
2. A hearing at which evidence is presented for the inmate's transfer and at which the inmate may present his own witnesses and cross-examine those called by the state.
3. An independent decisionmaker (not necessarily a judge), who must provide a written statement of the evidence and reasons for transfer.
4. Availability of "qualified and independent assistance" furnished by the state for inmates who are unable to furnish their own counsel (*Vitek v. Jones* 1980).

The extent to which these new protections have influenced the process is unclear. They are likely to screen out blatant abuses of the transfer process, although as noted earlier, such abuses are probably not common. But overall, it is doubtful that the process of transfers will be significantly influenced by the *Vitek* decision. Some prisons have developed their own mental health units, and some departments of correction have built their own security hospitals. Since these developments appear to be increasing, it is unclear whether a *Vitek*-type hearing is mandatory when transfers are made between units of a department of correction rather than between a department of correction and a department of mental health. Currently, transfers made within a department of correction appear largely to be accomplished by administrative directive and without formal hearings.

Legal Issues

Transferred inmates represent a class of mentally disordered offenders who are exceptions to the two assumptions usually made by the criminal justice system—*first*, that those who are sentenced to prison are unlikely to have severe mental disorders, and *second*, that conditions of imprisonment, while unpleasant, are sufficiently humane that the majority of offenders can endure them. If too many offenders turn out to be mentally ill when they reach prison, the fairness of the process that tried, convicted, and sentenced them can be questioned. If too many offenders become disordered as a result of confinement, the assumption that current conditions of imprisonment are humane can be challenged. To preserve the accuracy of its assumptions, the criminal justice system must deal with the issue of mental illness in prison by restricting the number of offenders who are formally defined as mentally disordered. Again, mentally disordered offenders turn out to be exceptions that prove the rule. In this section, I will argue that the assumptions that most offenders do not have mental disorders and can endure imprisonment without experiencing severe mental distress can be challenged.

Defining the Mentally Ill Offender

Most of the statutes concerning competency to stand trial and insanity do not include definitions of mental disorders or illnesses. Sex crime statutes either fail to define mental illness or are worded in such a manner that the existence of a mental disorder is simply inferred if deviant and repetitive sexual behavior is proven. Similarly, clear definitions of mental illness are lacking in most statutes authorizing transfers of disturbed inmates from prisons to mental hospitals. Even statutes authorizing civil commitment tend to dodge the issue of defining mental illness. A representative definition taken from the civil commitment statute of the State of North Carolina reads:

> An adult is mentally ill if he has an illness that so lessens his capacity to use self-control, judgment, and discretion in conducting his affairs and social relations as to make it necessary

or advisable for him to be under treatment, care, supervision, guidance, or control. (N.C. Gen. Sat. Section 122-36, 1979)

This statement emphasizes certain undesirable social characteristics that can be related to an illness and that it may be advisable to do something about; it does not, however, specifically define a mental illness.

In the absence of clear statutory definitions of mental disorder or illness, mental health professionals working in the legal setting have to rely on definitions created by their own profession. The official nomenclature presented in the *Diagnostic and Statistical Manual of Mental Disorders,* Third Edition (DSM-III), of the American Psychiatric Association (1980) does not use the term "mental illness" and describes all diagnosable conditions as mental disorders. The emphasis here is on identifying a clinically significant behavior or psychological syndrome that is typically associated with either painful symptoms (distress) or impairment in one or more important areas of functioning (disability). A qualification is typically made requiring inference that a behavioral, biological, or psychological basis to the disorder exists, and that the resulting disturbance is characterized by something more than a conflict between the individual and society.

The framers of DSM-III sought to include a wide number of impairments associated with distress or disability under a medical model. Although they tried to avoid the terms "illness" or "disease," they implied that mental disorders, like illnesses or diseases, are both preventable and treatable. By using the broad DSM-III criteria, psychiatrists and other mental health workers are given professional sanction to label a wide variety of behavior patterns, from drug dependence (including tobacco dependence) to mild depression and persistent patterns of maladjustment, as mental disorders. All behavior patterns that might trouble the individual or society are included, with the exception of unspecified forms of social deviancy.

Although mental health professionals are allowed to create their own definitions of mental illness or mental disorder, they cannot control or predict how society will respond to persons so diagnosed. Nor can they assume that the mentally ill will be treated with the same sympathy, compassion, and concern as the physically ill. One important variable in determining society's response to an illness is whether the cause of that disturbance is viewed as biological, i.e., involving some alteration in the anatomy or physiology of the afflicted person. In general, those who have disorders that have clear biological origins are treated most compassionately. In nonpsychiatric medicine, causation is viewed primarily as biological. The causes of most mental disorders, however, are unknown. (DSM-III is wisely silent on this issue.) Even when biological variations are discovered in those having psychiatric disorders, the extent to which these factors are causally related to the eventual clinical picture is unlikely to be clear. Mental disorders are powerfully influenced by environmental *as well as* biological variables.

The extent to which a disorder is considered to be biologically determined will exert a powerful influence on the manner in which those diagnosed as having that disorder will be held responsible for their symptoms. With rare exceptions, we do not blame people for symptoms associated with cancer or pneumonia; we view them as afflicted with a biological impairment and we excuse behavioral manifestations of their symptomatology. Mental disorders, however, are viewed more inconsistently. Sometimes the symptoms of mental disorder are viewed as beyond the disturbed person's power to control, and sometimes they are not. When evidence of biological dysfunction is clear, as is the case when individuals have organic brain disorders, we tend to excuse their behavior. In the absence of such evidence, society's response to the mentally disordered is likely to be inconsistent and ambivalent.

A critical and obvious determinant of society's response to the mentally disordered is the extent to which the behavioral manifestations of a particular disorder are troubling to society. Those who harm society are treated differently from those who do not, even if they receive the same psychiatric diagnosis. This is reflected in the different way diagnosis influences the treatment of patients in the free world, as opposed to the criminal justice system. In the free world, DSM-III diagnoses of either major or minor disorders (including personality disorders and anxiety disorders) usually result in consequences not too dissimilar from those following a diagnosis of a physical disorder. Persons diagnosed as having mental disorders are viewed, at least some of the time, as objects of concern and sympathy. They are afforded the opportunity for treatment by doctors and other mental health professionals. While society is uncertain about how responsible we should hold these people for their behavior, we do insure them, and, if they are hospitalized, their medical bills are often paid. If unable to work, they may be considered mentally disabled and be supported by government agencies.

The response of the criminal justice system to mental disorders is not nearly as compassionate. It considers only certain illnesses, such as schizophrenia, major affective disorders, or organic mental disorders (all of which have demonstrable or probable biological causation), as sufficiently severe to justify a compassionate or excusing response. Almost all other diagnoses elicit a different type of response. Minor disorders, such as anxiety reactions or somatoform disorders (disorders characterized by multiple complaints of physical distress without an organic basis), are often ignored. Disorders that may have a direct relation to the offense, such as a substance abuse disorder (e.g., alcoholism) or a personality disorder (e.g., antisocial personality disorder or narcissistic personality disorder), are either ignored or viewed as evidence of dangerousness; their existence may reflect adversely upon the offender. Once these so-called minor disorders are diagnosed, it is almost as if that part of the medical model that deals with the patient as an object of compassion rather than of blame becomes inoperative.

It can be argued, of course, that in the free world people are also ambivalent about whether individuals diagnosed as alcoholics or personality disorders should be viewed as "sick" or "bad." Angry and sometimes punitive responses toward these individuals are not uncommon, even in mental hospitals. Admittedly, the differences in compassion or punitiveness with which these individuals are greeted in the free world, as compared with the criminal justice system, is only one of degree. It is, nevertheless, a very critical difference. In the criminal justice system, individuals who are alcoholics or who have personality disorders are unlikely to be formally classified as mentally disordered offenders. Their diagnoses will have almost no influence on determining their competency, their insanity, or their need to be transferred to a hospital. Nor will diagnoses of alcoholism or personality disorder, made in the course of evaluating sex offenders, consistently influence whether they are sentenced to specialized treatment programs.

The practices of the criminal justice system are strengthened by the tendency of even the most eminent criminological researchers to accept the exclusion of alcoholism and personality disorders as mental disorders (Monahan and Steadman 1982). Such an exclusion is likely to be made on moral rather than on scientific principles. Acceptance or rejection of diagnostic categories on the basis of prevailing moral or social needs is hardly a new phenomenon in the medical and behavioral sciences. At various times physicians and behavioral scientists have allowed moral biases and social needs to compromise their commitment to scientific impartiality and have arbitrarily diagnosed those who do things society does not like as mentally ill (Halleck 1971).

I believe that similar biases have influenced both clinicians and researchers to discourage them from diagnosing criminals as mentally ill. Those who work in the criminal justice system blind themselves to the obvious impairments of many criminals, because recognizing their disabilities would require society to drastically reconsider its response to their behavior. A brief look at what has been learned about alcohol abuse and personality disorders would suggest that those who meet the DSM-III criteria for these conditions may well be seriously incapacitated individuals who are as logically placed in the mentally disordered category as those who are given more "serious" diagnoses.

Alcoholic Intoxication and Alcoholism

Alcoholic intoxication is classified as an organic mental disorder that may or may not be associated with the diagnoses of alcohol abuse and alcohol dependence. Ample evidence shows that it is a disorder closely associated with criminal behavior. The majority of apprehended felons are intoxicated at the time they commit a crime (Shupe 1954; Spieker and Sarver 1979). For violent crimes like homicide, that percentage varies between 63 percent and 83 percent (McDonald 1961). The existence of such a correlation does not in itself explain how alcoholic intoxication is related to criminal behavior (Collins 1981). It is possible that offenders may become intoxicated in order to free themselves of inhibitions that might have prevented them from committing crimes. Or, for some offenders, intoxication and criminal conduct may simply be unrelated events. It can even be argued that extreme intoxication might prevent certain crimes by rendering some individuals so stuporous that they are unable to carry them out.

Finally, the extent to which intoxication increases an offender's likelihood of being apprehended is unclear. In some instances, intoxication may have been a more important factor in apprehension than in causation. Even with these qualifications, however, it appears that among the majority of offenders who are caught, it is possible to trace a direct pattern of causation between intoxication and crime. Intoxicated offenders are impaired in their capacity to perceive alternatives and to perceive and evaluate the risks and benefits of a crime. Many crimes would thus not have been committed *but for* the offender's intoxication.

Those who are intoxicated inflict this condition upon themselves. While intoxicated, however, they are biologically impaired and their capacities are likely to be less than those of sober offenders. To the extent that alcohol-abusing offenders retain a propensity to become intoxicated when released, they may also be considered more likely to repeat their crimes than other offenders. Given these realities, it would seem that a diagnosis of intoxication at the time of a crime would have a major impact on the offender's disposition. In practice, such a diagnosis has little influence on judgments regarding culpability or treatment, and it is not consistently weighed in making judgments of dangerousness.

The criminal justice system is especially concerned that intoxication not be viewed as an exculpatory factor, in order to discourage persons from becoming intoxicated before a crime in order to avoid punishment. However, proof of intoxication at the time of the crime is rarely sufficient to allow the offender to completely avoid punishment. While intoxication can be a mitigating factor when the death penalty is at issue, or may be a consideration in determining if an offender had the specific intent to commit a particular crime, it is otherwise unlikely to influence criminal liability. Similarly, a history of intoxication does not influence disposition of offenders in prison. Those offenders who define their tendency to become intoxicated as a manifestation of an emotional problem are given the opportunity to seek help through such organizations as Alcoholics Anonymous. Their treatment, however, is not mandated.

The majority of apprehended offenders, in addition to having a history of being intoxicated at the time of a crime, also have a history of chronic alcohol abuse (Guze et al. 1968). The extent of such abuse is often sufficient to permit diagnosis, using DSM-III criteria, of an alcohol abuse disorder or an alcohol dependence disorder. In the free world, alcoholism is considered a disease. (According to a recent Gallup poll, 80 percent of Americans now believe that alcoholism is a disease.) While this response has developed slowly and ambivalently, it has considerable scientific foundation. Impressive evidence has shown that susceptibility to alcohol abuse is inherited (Cloninger et al. 1981). Moreover, alcoholism is frequently associated with other major disturbances such as affective disorders (Andreasen and Winokur 1979). Biological differences between alcoholics and social drinkers in their responsivity to alcohol have also been demonstrated (Lender and Martin 1982). Over time, those who are diagnosed as alcoholics suffer greatly and are seriously impaired in their capacity to function as law-abiding citizens. The disorder is likely to have played some role in their crimes and will probably increase the likelihood that they will commit crimes in the future.

The relationship of chronic alcoholism to crime is just as complex as the relationship of acute intoxication to crime. The coexistence of alcoholism and criminality may in some individuals be unrelated. But alcoholism can favor criminal conduct, or repetitive criminal conduct may make a person more likely to turn to alcohol. On the other hand, both alcoholism and criminality can be related to a third factor, while chronic alcoholism itself may so impair some individuals that they lack the mental or physical capacities to commit a crime. As is the case with intoxication, however, these qualifications do not negate the reality that, in a majority of cases, a causal linkage can be defined between alcohol abuse and the eventual commission of a crime.

Overall, a diagnosis of alcoholism has little more influence on the disposition of offenders than a diagnosis of intoxication at the time of the crime. It is almost never an exculpatory factor. And while alcoholism may be considered in assessing future dangerousness, offenders who are viewed as alcoholics are treated only on a voluntary basis.

Personality Disorders

Personality traits are enduring patterns of perceiving, relating to, and thinking about the environment and oneself. When individuals demonstrate these traits, when the traits are maladaptive, and when they cause either significant impairment in social or occupational functioning or subjective distress, they are diagnosed as having personality disorders. There are four classes of personality disorders, characterized by dramatic, emotional, or erratic behavior, which are often grouped together. These are the histrionic, the narcissistic, the antisocial, and the borderline personality disorders. Each of these disorders can be extremely incapacitating. Some evidence exists of biological dysfunction and extreme psychological impairment associated with each category. Many criminal offenders fit the criteria for one or more of these personality disorders (Guze 1976). Greatest attention, however, has been focused on the relationship of the antisocial personality (often called psychopathic or sociopathic personality) to criminal behavior.

For at least two centuries now, many mental health profession-als have argued that a group of individuals can be identified who habitually fail to adhere to the rules of society, and who are so different from the rest of us that they should be considered men-tally disordered (Cleckley 1955). While these persons do not always appear to suffer as much as those we think of as having tradi-tional mental disorders, they are, nevertheless, substantially dis-abled in their capacity to adjust to society. They tend to be self-defeating, unwilling or unable to form successful interpersonal re-lationships, relatively unresponsive to punitive sanctions, and a source of constant distress to the community. While their defect is often viewed as a moral one, many theories have been proposed suggesting that their moral incapacity is related either to highly deleterious learning experiences in early life and/or to a maladap-tive biological variation (Mednick and Volavka 1980).

Theories as to the nature of the biological variation in these persons are of special interest here. They cover a wide range of scientific validity or sophistication. Most of the early theories were based on armchair speculation or on clinical observation of small groups of subjects. Recently, more careful studies have pro-vided evidence that persons we ordinarily think of as psychopathic or sociopathic differ from other people in being less responsive to external stimuli and in having more difficulty developing condi-tioned responses (Mednick and Volavka 1980). While the theories of crime and psychopathy that have developed out of this research must be viewed cautiously, when they are considered in light of evidence showing some genetic basis for habitual criminality, it becomes reasonable to argue that there appears to be a class of in-dividuals who inherit minor neurological variations that ultimately make them more susceptible to criminal behavior (Mednick and Hutchings 1977).

In current psychiatric nomenclature, those previously diagnosed as suffering from psychopathic or sociopathic personalities are now diagnosed as having antisocial personality disorders. The criteria for diagnosis have also changed. The older diagnoses of psychopathic or sociopathic personality were based largely on in-ferences about the patient's lack of guilt or conscience. The mod-ern diagnosis of antisocial personality is based on more observable criteria, such as antisocial behavior in childhood, habitual law-breaking, and vocational and interpersonal maladjustments. How-ever, the percentage of habitual criminals who fit these criteria remains unclear. Nevertheless, the experience of those who work in correctional institutions would suggest that this percentage would be extremely high, perhaps over 50 percent (Rennie 1978). In fact, if the DSM-III diagnosis of antisocial personality disorder were accepted as a legitimate disorder, the majority of incarcerated offenders could be viewed as mentally ill.

It may be useful to pause briefly and acknowledge the confusion pervading this issue and how easy it is to become trapped in circular thinking. If we say that those who meet the criteria of antisocial personality disorder have a mental disorder and that those criteria simply define habitual criminality, we may be doing nothing more than labeling habitual criminality a disease. Furthermore, the studies suggesting a biological basis for this disorder have been conducted on populations defined by a variety of imprecise criteria. Some involved persons who fit the older criteria of sociopathy and psychopathy, some were done on individuals diagnosed as antisocial personalities, and some involved habitual criminals who had received no psychiatric diagnosis.

In spite of all the circular thinking and confusion in the field, certain conclusions can still be drawn. A substantial number of offenders may have some genetic predisposition to crime. This same group may have minor variations in their autonomic nervous systems that impair their capacity to learn and enjoy law-abiding behavior. While the developers of DSM-III may have contributed to our confusion by defining the antisocial personality disorder in terms associated with habitual criminality, it is likely that offenders who receive this diagnosis will belong to a group who may have some biological impairment. This impairment may diminish their capacity to make law-abiding adjustments and thus can be considered a causal factor in understanding their past criminality. Also, its presence may increase the likelihood of future criminality.

Currently, the criminal justice system does not respond to a diagnosis of antisocial personality disorder as though it were a real illness. Rather, it responds in two essentially punitive ways. First, the diagnosis is used to imply that no "real" illness is present. When a psychiatric report lists no diagnosis other than antisocial personality disorder, it almost always negates a finding of incompetency or insanity and will usually discourage a mitigating or merciful disposition. Second, the diagnosis may be used to imply dangerousness. In sentencing procedures, a diagnosis of antisocial personality disorder is likely to be viewed as an aggravating factor that justifies greater punishment. The diagnosis of antisocial personality is almost never associated with recommendations for treatment. Nor are individuals with this diagnosis likely to be treated in prison, unless they are placed in special segregated programs for "troublemakers." In general, the manner in which the criminal justice system currently responds to diagnoses of antisocial personality makes for a somewhat paradoxical situation: a diagnostic category that is probably associated with an organic disability is used to justify retribution rather than compassion.

While the relationship of narcissistic, histrionic, and borderline personality disorders to crime has never been systematically studied, correctional psychiatrists have sometimes observed a high incidence of symptoms characteristic of these disorders among offenders (Vaillant and Perry 1980). Indeed, it would be reasonable to assume that these highly disabling conditions have some causal link to criminal behavior. The evidence that histrionic, narcissistic, and borderline personality disorders are associated with some degree of biological impairment is moderately persuasive (Siever 1983). These individuals are highly susceptible to a variety of forms of anxiety and depression. They appear to suffer much more than those who have antisocial personality disorders, and sometimes the criminal justice system responds to them in a beneficent manner. When these personality disorders are associated with memory loss, fugue states, or other dissociative phenomena, such as the presence of multiple personalities, they may be considered in assessing competency or criminal liability. Sometimes sex offenders are given these diagnoses to justify their specialized treatment. Most of the time, however, the criminal justice system does not alter its usual practices in responding to offenders diagnosed as having any type of personality disorder.

Mental Retardation

The idiosyncratic responsiveness of the criminal justice system to psychiatric diagnosis is also evident in its treatment of mentally retarded offenders. In the most frequently quoted survey of the intellectual capacities of incarcerated offenders, 9.5 percent were found to have IQ scores below 70 (Brown and Courtless 1968). It is likely (but not certain) that offenders found to be moderately to severely retarded (IQs below 50) are diverted from the criminal process as incompetent to stand trial, while those within the mildly retarded range (IQs 50 to 70) are usually treated like ordinary criminals. Although this group is characterized as mildly retarded, their educational, social, and vocational skills are generally so deficient that they need special guidance and assistance to make a satisfactory adjustment in the free world. Many of them also experience extreme difficulties in adjusting to the correctional setting.

The relationship of mental retardation to crime raises the same issues encountered in considering the relationship of alcoholism to crime. Although the case for direct causation is probably weaker, we know that mental retardation may be a critical factor in at least some crimes. We also know that, in many instances, the limited capacities of retarded individuals are determined by biological rather than environmental variations. As is the case with diagnoses of alcohol or personality disorders, a diagnosis of mental retardation might elicit compassionate and exculpatory responses in the free world but be largely ignored by the criminal justice system.

Mental Health in the Prison Environment

To the extent that mental disorders are determined by unfavorable environments, the institutional correctional system must be viewed as playing a significant role in creating, perpetuating, or aggravating such disorders. Imprisonment imposes many stresses upon offenders, usually far in excess of those that might result if the only punishment were deprivation of liberty. Prisons in most countries are not simply places of restraint. They are institutions that impose unusual psychological pain upon their occupants. Deprivations, mortifications, and abuses that are much in excess of those required to keep them from harming society are regularly inflicted upon prisoners. The eminent psychiatrist Karl Menninger has argued that if one were to assess all of the harm imposed upon criminals as a consequence of their punishment and compare it with all the harm those same offenders have imposed upon society, incarcerated criminals may well have suffered more than their victims (Menninger 1968). The level of pain currently inflicted on offenders is much greater than that proposed by utilitarian advocates of deterrence theory, who believe that punishment should be just severe enough to deter, or by the advocates of "just deserts," who believe that the amount of harm inflicted on offenders should be proportional to the amount of harm they have inflicted upon society.

The creation of a high rate of mental disorder may be one of the natural consequences of a criminal justice system that relies too heavily on harsh conditions of prolonged imprisonment as its major response to the offender. In the process of punishing offenders, the system deprives them of gratifications that may be viewed as essential to the maintenance of mental health. Some of the gratifications universally assumed to be essential to mental health will be listed here along with a brief commentary on the extent to which they are currently gratified in prisons.

1. *Intimacy.* The opportunity and capacity to form gratifying interpersonal relationships is for most people an essential condition of human happiness. Some people may survive with comfort in isolation from other humans, but this requires an abundance of other reinforcers in their environment, such as animals, access to natural beauty, or interesting activities. The commonest precipitant of mental illness in the free world is probably the stress associated with loss of intimacy. In prison, the offender is denied access to loved ones. Intimacy with other prisoners or correctional offers is discouraged or viewed as a form of deviant conduct. Gratifying activities that can be conducted in isolation from others are few or nonexistent.

2. *Influence.* All individuals try to retain some control over how they interact with others. They are gratified when their behavior elicits predictable and desired responses in others. Prison inmates have little power, except over other weaker inmates. They have little influence on their day-to-day activity, which is largely ordained for them by their keepers. Until their sentence expires or their parole date is reached, they can do almost nothing about their future, except try to escape or write writs of appeal.

3. *Autonomy.* The capacity to feel that one can make choices is an essential aspect of human existence. Those who experience their choices as arbitrarily limited experience themselves as oppressed. Prisoners are automatically deprived of many choices by virtue of being incarcerated, but they could, in theory, still have varying degrees of freedom within the institution. Conceivably, prisons could be developed in which offenders had a wide variety of choices involving their daily activities. The modern tendency, however, has been to create prisons in which offenders have as little autonomy as possible. The time they get up in the morning, what they eat, who they see, the kind of work they do, and when they go to bed are all rigidly controlled. Such a regime may be tolerable to passive individuals who have given up all hope of autonomy, but for most offenders who still see themselves as individuals with the capacity to make choices, it is a major source of deprivation and pain.

4. *Physical Activity.* A certain amount of activity in the form of work or creative recreation is an essential aspect of human contentedness, and in this area the prison directly stifles human

needs. Little useful work is available in most prisons. There may even be stringent limits on the opportunity for physical exercise. A certain amount of art and writing is fostered by the prison milieu, but such creativity is characteristic only of those prisoners who have unusual strength of purpose or talents.

5. *Privacy.* While individuals need to relate to others, they also occasionally need to be alone. However, this may be impossible in the correctional setting. Overcrowding makes even a few moments of daily privacy a luxury in all but a few institutions. The only time prisoners are likely to be alone is when they are being punished in an isolation unit. Here most of them experience massive sensory deprivation, which is so painful that it negates the benefits of privacy. In most prisons, even the simple pleasure of enjoying brief periods of silence is unavailable. Prisons are noisy places filled with the unpleasant sounds of screams, tears, clanging doors, and machinery. Even at night, silence is a luxury and peaceful sleep a rarity.

In addition to creating stress by deprivation, prison creates stress by threatening the safety of inmates. Inmates who are not predators live in constant fear of sexual or other types of physical assault. Even predators must worry that a stronger force will emerge and they will become prey. Prisoners in some institutions resemble soldiers on a battlefield. They are chronically alert to the fear of attack, live in a state of apprehension, and are prone to suffer the bodily and mental ills of those who have been in a combat zone too long.

It could be argued that the conditions I have described here, including the lack of influence, freedom, or privacy, might also describe certain slum or ghetto communities in our society, and that individuals who come from such communities would be less likely to view imprisonment as a major punishment. One weakness of this argument is that ghettos are also highly stressful environments whose inhabitants experience more suffering and mental illness than residents of less stressful communities. We would not wish to justify ghettos any more than we would wish to justify bad prisons. A more important counterargument could be made by comparing the degree of suffering experienced in prison with that in the slums. No matter how bad life in the slums may be, its inhabitants are still free human beings whose opportunities for intimacy, influence, freedom, physical activity, and privacy far exceed those available to prisoners.

Whether by design or accident, prisons are superb breeding grounds for mental illness. Thus, we should never be surprised when offenders become mentally ill in the course of their punishment. What is more surprising, however, is that so many survive the ordeal.

Individual Responsivity to Prison-Inflicted Pain

In spite of the consistent oppressiveness of the prison environment, individual variations among prisoners are such that they may respond to it quite differently. At one extreme, a certain number of individuals, already mentally disturbed on entering prison, are highly vulnerable to the stresses of prison and quickly become mentally ill. At the other extreme, a certain number of individuals seem to comfortably endure the prison environment. The latter group forms a small but fascinating minority. Often, they are persons who have known very harsh conditions on the outside. For this group, the experience of loss following imprisonment may not be overwhelming. They may also be helped by having a flexible sexual orientation. Some of the most comfortable prisoners are homosexuals who are also capable of defending themselves. They, at least, are not deprived of the sexual aspect of intimacy and can avoid assault. Also, a certain number of people have exceptional capacities to endure a lack of intimacy, physical activity, influence, or freedom. Some of these individuals appear to be able to tolerate prolonged periods of isolation or segregation without experiencing long-term ill effects. It is conceivable that these individuals have significant neurological variations that are not adaptive in the free world but which enable them to comfortably endure a degree of stress in prison that normal individuals could not tolerate.

The majority of offenders suffer through their imprisonment but are never considered mentally ill. Their capacity to resist assuming the sick role or its involuntary imposition is determined by a variety of individual and environmental variables. As a general rule, a past history of interpersonal and occupational achievement, plus a past history of relative freedom from anxiety or depression, augurs for a painful but relatively successful prison adjustment. Certain circumstances in the correctional environment, such as the availability of close friends, may make a difference. The continued support of friends and families on the outside or the capacity to develop a more spiritual view of life also helps some inmates endure their ordeal.

A final but critical consideration in determining whether an offender comes to be seen as mentally disordered is the clinical sensitivity of the staff. In some institutions, inmates can be severely depressed or even psychotic without anybody's noticing their condition. Or, inmates may be aware of intense personal suffering but feel that they should cover it up because more harm than help would come from complaining of symptoms. I am never surprised, when visiting a prison and being asked to interview prisoners described as typical or as "troublemakers," to discover that they are blatantly psychotic. Even a minimal empathic inquiry into their mental status reveals what is often extraordinary pathology.

Whether we label it as mental illness or not, mental suffering is the norm in our prisons. Most inmates survive in a state of chronic anxiety and depression. Many are dysfunctional. Even those who appear to survive the experience may continue to have symptoms such as anxiety and depression for many years after release. If we were objective in considering the mental condition of all prisoners and did not focus only upon the few who are so disturbed as to need transfer to a hospital, we could not hold to the belief that the latter few are exceptional. Society's assumption that imprisonment is an experience that can be endured by the majority of prisoners without becoming psychologically damaged is untenable. Given the state of our prisons, the individual who survives imprisonment psychologically undamaged is the true exception to the norm.

This is an appropriate place to note that consideration of the differences in individual responsiveness to imprisonment also exposes major sources of unfairness in our current emphasis on retributive justice. When the courts impose sentences, the severity of punishment is usually measured by the length of imprisonment, not by the actual degree of suffering inflicted upon the offender. The psychological issue of the offender's probable response to punishment is usually ignored. One need only spend a few minutes interviewing a random group of prisoners to grasp the fallacy of this approach. Responses to punishment may vary depending on the socioeconomic status, the past learning experiences, the age, the health, or the nervous systems of offenders. Three days in prison will be as painful to some individuals as 3 years for others.

Clinical Issues

The prevalence of mental disorder in prison and the tendency of prisons to perpetuate it pose unusual problems for clinicians.

(Some of these will be considered in subsequent chapters.) Perhaps the most obvious is that the need for clinical services in the correctional setting is always likely to exceed the supply. The tendency of departments of correction to minimize the prevalence of mental disorder in prisons is reflected in budgeting for clinical positions. There has probably never been a correctional institution in the United States that has had an adequate clinical staff. As a rule, clinicians who are both compassionate and competent quickly become overworked. Even inmates who may have good reason to hide their disabilities are likely to seek the help of good clinicians if they are available. Competent clinicians are in the position of having to make triage-type decisions on a regular basis. They must decide if services are to be provided by considering the severity of the offenders' disorders, their immediate needs to adjust to the prison milieu, their capacities to have a favorable short-term response to treatment, and their likelihood of making a favorable long-term adjustment in the free world.

A different kind of problem of clinical judgment arises when the actual decision for transfer must be made. The clinician will encounter many offenders who could probably benefit from treatment in a security hospital. Transfer, however, cannot be determined solely by the immediate needs of offenders. Clinicians also must consider the long-term consequences of transfer, the formidable disadvantages of which have already been noted. In dealing with offenders who are especially likely to respond adversely to the stigmatization of being labeled mentally ill, clinicians may find it beneficial not to transfer them but to find some way to treat them in the correctional environment (Thurrell et al. 1965). This approach diminishes the likelihood that offenders will be tempted to adopt the role of a mental patient. It allows offenders to retain whatever ties they have to others in prison and gives them an opportunity to deal directly with the stresses of imprisonment that may have engendered their disorder. The advantages of this approach are similar to those for mentally ill patients in the free world when they are treated in their own communities in lieu of hospitalization.

Another difficult problem for clinicians is that they must attempt to treat mental disorders in an environment where the levels of stress make the mental condition of offenders worse. Clinicians can do little about these conditions, and if they try too hard to modify them they risk losing credibility with other correctional workers. In addition, clinicians must be especially cognizant of the mental health values they must utilize in attempting to help offenders. While in most clinical settings behavior such as assertiveness, self-disclosure, and honesty is believed to be highly correlated with mental health, in correctional settings, this may not be true. Sometimes it is adaptive for offenders to be withdrawn, dishonest, or even antisocial. Clinicians must find some means of modifying their usual clinical values. They sometimes must be less concerned with the offenders' short-term welfare than with the ultimate goal of helping offenders survive the ordeal of imprisonment with the least harm to themselves or to the institution.

Emerging Legal Issues

While recent litigation protecting the procedural rights of offenders facing transfer to security hospitals has received a great deal of attention from legal scholars, it is doubtful that such litigation has had a meaningful impact on more than a few inmates. As noted previously, many transferred offenders are simply retained under the jurisdiction of a department of corrections and probably do not receive hearings anyway. It is also likely that the majority of offenders who are emotionally disturbed are willing to receive treatment and do not resist transfer. Finally, even if offenders are transferred against their will, there is reason to doubt that the possible harm to them from transfer would outweigh the potential benefits. All these reasons suggest little cause to anticipate further legal change focused on protection of the offender in the transfer process.

The issue of transfer does, however, call our attention to the entire question of mental illness in prisons and the adequacy with which it is currently treated. It could be argued that prisoners are entitled to full medical services and have a right to mental health treatment. Thus far, the courts have not been overly generous in defining the extent of services constitutionally mandated for prisoners (*Bowring v. Godwin* 1977); (*Estelle v. Gamble* 1976). Nevertheless, exceptions may be created for certain classes of prisoners. Offenders adjudicated as "guilty but mentally ill," for example, are by statute entitled to some type of mental health treatment while in prison. The Supreme Court of Michigan has recently ordered the provision of addition mental health services for GBMI offenders in that state's prisons.

CHAPTER 7

Practical Issues: Assessment,
Disposition, and Treatment

IN ADDITION TO SERVING the judicial system by assessing such issues as pretrial competency, insanity, and dangerousness, mental health clinicians manage and treat mentally disordered offenders on a day-to-day basis. The circumstances under which assessment and treatment are conducted are quite different for mentally disordered offenders as compared with most mentally disturbed individuals. Assessment may be made more difficult because of limited resources or resistant attitudes on the part of offenders. Therapeutic interventions must often be tailored to the correctional environment. Sometimes, traditional treatment approaches have to be modified because of lack of adequate resources. Or, they may be modified on the basis of a belief that mentally ill offenders require different forms of treatment than other patients.

Problems in Evaluation

The Appropriateness of Referrals

The quality and usefulness of assessment and subsequent treatment are in large part determined by the appropriateness of referrals for evaluation. Inappropriate referrals for evaluation of competency to stand trial are relatively frequent. In dealing with incompetent offenders, security hospitals have no control over the admissions process. The courts have total discretion to determine who will be evaluated, and when and where the evaluation will be done. Not infrequently, the courts request evaluations of competency for a variety of reasons other than an actual need to determine the offender's capacity to proceed in the criminal process.

Defense attorneys and judges may initiate competency evaluations to help determine whether the offender was insane at the time of the crime or was in a state of mind that would negate the *mens rea* of the crime. Or, the request for an incompetency evaluation may be simply an attempt to gain psychological data that the judge might later consider in the process of sentencing. These uses of the forensic hospital are not especially troubling as long as evaluators and offenders have a clear sense of the issues actually being considered. A more troubling practice, which is clearly an abuse of the evaluation process, involves sending individuals to maximum security hospitals for a competency evaluation when the court's real intention is to ensure that these persons are temporarily incarcerated and, perhaps, treated. With the advent of stricter criteria for involuntary civil commitment, a certain number of highly disturbed individuals who used to be kept in public mental hospitals are now free to roam the streets (Chase 1973). Some of them are nuisances to the community, engaging in offenses such as trespassing, disturbing the peace, or petty theft. Because of the minor nature of their offenses, the criminal justice system is often unwilling to imprison them. A not infrequent solution these days is to arrest them on a minor charge and then have them sent to a security hospital for evaluation of competency to stand trial. Since the evaluation period at these facilities can be as long as 15 to 60 days, the defendant is at least temporarily removed from the community.

There is something absurd about shipping persons hundreds of miles to evaluate their competency to stand trial for crimes such as "walking on a rail" or "failure to pay a toll" (P. Dietz, personal communication, 1983). The evaluation becomes an excuse to keep the offender in a rather costly and often oppressive custodial setting. But institutions differ in their approach to these referrals. Some, in addition to going through the charade of evaluating competency, accept the responsibility of providing the treatment denied in the community. They use all forms of psychiatric treatment, including pharmacotherapy, counseling, and consultation to community agencies, to help these defendants make less troublesome adjustments in their communities. Other institutions simply endure the situation. They go through the motions of evaluation, offer perfunctory treatment, and return defendants to court as competent to stand trial as soon as possible. At this point, the court usually drops charges and releases them.

Availability of Data and Resources

Even when referrals are appropriate, the evaluation of mentally disordered offenders is often a more difficult task than evaluation of ordinary patients. A major problem is the availability of objective history. In the ordinary clinical setting, the evaluator usually has access to old records, hospital reports, and family members or friends of the patient who may be reliable reporters. Those sent to a forensic hospital for assessment of competency, however, may arrive with nothing more than a court order. The evaluator may be informed only that the defendant has been charged with a specific crime. Even police reports may be lacking. If the institution to which the defendant is sent is located some distance from the defendant's home, there may be no possibility of obtaining objective history from friends or family. The evaluator can look for old hospital and prison records, but this is a time-consuming enterprise, and it may take weeks or months before such data become available. (The situation is not as difficult when the offender has already been convicted and the evaluator is making recommendations regarding sentencing or transfer. Here, at least, a good possibility exists that a presentence report prepared by a probation officer will be available.)

Historical data can, in theory, be obtained from the defendant. Many defendants, however, are not accurate reporters of their past behavior. Even if their memories and thought processes are relatively intact, they are unlikely to be very objective. Offenders who are even minimally capable of comprehending reality know that the forensic evaluation will influence their disposition. This knowledge will influence their behavior during a psychiatric examination. If charged with very serious crimes and if faced with long sentences, offenders may want to accentuate qualities that would make them look incompetent. If charged with crimes carrying light penalties, they may try to look as competent as they can. Where acquittal by reason of insanity holds out the possibility of early release, defendants may perceive a need to present themselves in as disturbed a manner as possible. On the other hand, defendants being examined for possible commitment to an indeterminate sex offender's program may wish to deny any manifestation of pathology. Defendants being evaluated for possible transfer, depending upon their assessment of the personal advantages and disadvantages involved, will either exaggerate or minimize their disturbances.

The degree of accuracy with which defendants present their

history is, of course, determined by many factors, including the degree of rapport they develop with the examiner. Sometimes a skilled interviewer can learn a great deal from a defensive patient (Halleck 1967). As a general rule, however, the examiner is at risk of obtaining a distorted picture of the patient's past history. If and when an objective history is obtained, it usually is at some variance with the patient's version of the same events and will reveal more evidence of mental disability or previous criminality than the defendant was willing to acknowledge.

The diagnostic process in a jail, prison, or security hospital may also be compromised by the lack of availability of important psychological and laboratory tests. In most prisons and even in many maximum security hospitals, it is difficult to obtain psychological testing other than for intelligence. Sophisticated neuropsychological testing, which is very helpful in assessing the cognitive capacities of mentally disordered offenders (who are highly prone to abuse their brains by using drugs and are at high risk of getting into physical altercations where they may suffer head injuries), is rarely available. Projective testing may be available in programs that deal with mentally disordered sex offenders, but it may be difficult to obtain for other offenders. The availability of electroencephalograms, CAT scans, or laboratory procedures such as thyroid function studies or the dexamethazone suppression test is quite variable. A few institutions have arrangements with community hospitals that make these procedures available. Using outside facilities, however, is expensive, requires time and personnel, and puts some strain on security needs. When the indications for using expensive laboratory tests are not compelling, the tests are likely to be deleted from the evaluation process.

To the extent that objective history is unavailable and customary diagnostic procedures are not used, evaluations in the forensic setting tend to lack the validity of other mental health examinations. In an occasional case, where the crime is sensational or the defendant wealthy, very comprehensive workups may be done. But in most instances, the forensic evaluation is not as good as ordinary mental health evaluations performed in private or even public settings.

Professional Role Problems

The process of evaluating and treating mentally disordered offenders is almost always influenced by shortages of professional staff. When adequate staff is not available, evaluations tend to be brief and unreliable and treatment is less effective. The roles that various professions assume in the diagnostic and treatment process also change. In most public or private hospital settings, psychiatrists assume major responsibility for managing patients, prescribing drugs, and psychotherapy. In correctional or forensic settings, psychiatrists must spend a good deal of time preparing for courtroom testimony. Their evaluations may be directed more toward legal than therapeutic issues, and they may have little involvement in the therapeutic process. Much of the day-to-day administration and provision of counseling or psychotherapy in institutions that treat mentally disordered offenders is conducted by psychologists and social workers, who are somewhat easier to recruit into the correctional setting than psychiatrists. The relatively expensive time of psychiatrists tends to be reserved for tasks at which they are especially skilled or for which the law requires a licensed physician. Psychiatrists, therefore, may have little involvement in the process of treatment other than the management of pharmacotherapy.

While this distribution of labor may be efficient, it creates certain problems for all involved. The best trained psychiatrists will quickly become discontent when their diagnostic work is not integrated with treatment and they cannot use psychotherapeutic intervention or manage patients. While psychologists and social workers may welcome the opportunity to be administrators and therapists, they will usually come to resent a situation in which they do the most critical work but are paid half as much as the physician. It can be argued that a similar problem of discontent with professional roles exists in most public mental health centers. The situation in corrections, however, has more serious consequences. Recruiting any professional to work in the grim and frightening correctional setting is especially difficult. If professionals become discontent in the correctional or forensic setting, they will quickly depart to take better jobs. The turnover of certain professionals, particularly psychiatrists, tends to be high, and those who can be recruited are not likely to be the most skilled.

Treatment Issues: General Problems

The Meaning of Treatment in the Criminal Justice System

The term "treatment" usually connotes benevolent efforts to help an individual. However, in the criminal justice system (and also in dealing with involuntarily committed patients), the term may represent interventions that are used primarily to further the needs of society. Three models of intervention found in the criminal justice system, while based on different objectives, can all be viewed as models of treatment.

1. It can be assumed that the mental disorders of some offenders have a causal influence on their criminal behavior. In such instances, beneficent objectives and efforts to protect society by rehabilitating offenders are compatible. Both offenders and society are likely to benefit if treatment is successful.

The concordance of individual and societal goals is most likely to arise in dealing with offenders found not guilty by reason of insanity. Here, a crime has been adjudicated to be distinctly related to a mental disorder. Presumably, treatment of persons who have such illnesses should prevent their subsequent criminality. Mental health specialists who treat these patients can, in theory, help their patients while providing substantial benefits to society. A similar situation may at times exist in dealing with mentally disordered sex offenders or occasionally with offenders designated as antisocial personalities. In these cases, offenders are usually designated mentally disordered on the basis of behavior closely related to their crime. It is sometimes assumed that treatment will relieve these persons of whatever suffering may be caused by their disorder, at the same time that it diminishes their propensity to crime.

2. The mental disorders of some offenders may be assumed to have no relationship to their criminal behavior and may not even have been present until they entered the criminal justice process. Treating this kind of mental disorder is not likely to have an effect upon subsequent criminal conduct. When the mental disorders of such persons are treated, the motivations of therapists are in large part beneficent. The emphasis is on relieving the suffering of offenders or on helping them adjust to imprisonment. No assumption can be made that treatment will be rehabilitative.

Intervention that is not intended to rehabilitate is most likely to be used in dealing with offenders who become mentally ill in prison and have to be treated in special units or transferred to hospitals. Probably the majority of offenders receiving treatment in the criminal justice system are not viewed as likely to be rehabilitated as a result of treatment.

3. The most intriguing model of intervention in the criminal justice setting involves the use of techniques that are generally ef-

fective with clients who may not have a clearly defined mental disorder. In these cases, the concern is only with rehabilitation. (The many meanings of the term "rehabilitation" will be considered in the chapter on ethics. As used here, rehabilitation simply means doing something to offenders to reduce the likelihood that they would commit crimes if they were free.) Under this model of intervention, the treater need not be concerned with the well-being of those who are treated.

In the criminal justice setting, traditional psychiatric treatments, such as psychotherapy, behavior therapy, or pharmacotherapy, may be used to control the behavior of offenders who are viewed as having antisocial tendencies but not necessarily as mentally ill. Such treatment is usually involuntary, or offenders may "volunteer" for treatment with some coercion. The purpose is usually long-term behavioral change. Treatment for "rehabilitation only" purposes is possible, because certain interventions can influence behavior irrespective of whether such behavior is viewed as an aspect of a mental disorder. If a criminal behavior pattern is changed as a result of a clinical intervention (such as drug therapy), it does not follow that the criminal behavior was a manifestation of a mental disorder. It is possible to alter the bodily responses or learning pattern of any person, using drugs, behavior modification, or certain forms of psychotherapy. In theory, clinical intervention could even be used to make people more, rather than less, antisocial. The use of psychiatric treatments to rehabilitate or control offenders whose mental abnormality is in doubt has important ethical implications that will be considered in the next chapter.

Problems in Determining the Locus of Treatment

The decision to transfer a prisoner from one setting to another must usually be sanctioned by mental health professionals. The cost-benefit analysis a clinician makes in initiating or approving a transfer decision is somewhat different from that undertaken in ordinary practice. The needs of the institutions involved, as well as the offender's probable response to highly unusual environments, have to be considered.

The transferring institution gains certain advantages in getting rid of emotionally troubled offenders. Their illnesses may make them more vulnerable to predatory inmates or more dangerous to peaceful inmates. They are also at risk of hurting themselves. At the same time, any transfer of an inmate out of the ordinary prison population is not entirely without cost to the prison administration. A certain amount of administrative paperwork always accompanies the transfer procedure. In some instances, staff must be available for judicial proceedings. Prison administrators must also be concerned with the possibility that inmates will simulate or exaggerate mental disorder to enjoy whatever benefits might accrue if they are placed in a different environment. If too many prisoners used illness behaviors in a manipulative manner to gain transfers, prisons would be unmanageable.

Some of the advantages offenders may enjoy as a result of transfer, such as the opportunity to receive treatment in a safer and less oppressive environment, were noted in chapter 6. It may also be noted that some inmates recognize that they will have more power on a hospital unit. It is not uncommon for an inmate who is frequently victimized in the prison setting to turn into a predator in the hospital setting. Prisoners may also perceive certain advantages to adopting a sick role. In addition to receiving increased attention, those labeled as ill may, even in security hospitals, sometimes claim nonresponsibility for engaging in behaviors that would elicit punishment in most environments. Finally, inmates may enjoy a transfer simply because they are bored with prison life and desire a change.

At the same time, inmates recognize special risks to transfer, such as compromising the possibility of parole, loss of "good time," loss of civil rights, or stigmatization. The risk of being labeled mentally ill is an especially powerful one for offenders. Prisoners may be even less tolerant of the mentally ill than the rest of society. Inmates transferred to a hospital unit tend to be labeled as "bugs" or "psychos" by other inmates, and their status in the prison hierarchy may be permanently impaired. Some inmates will also find day-to-day contact with other mentally disordered offenders oppressive.

Another risk of transfer for offenders, which they are not likely to consider but which cannot be ignored by the clinician, is that, once they are in the hospital setting, they will learn to accept the sick role. Offenders who have serious personality disorders of the antisocial, histrionic, narcissistic, or borderline type tend to escalate their symptomatology, particularly symptoms of depression and anxiety, in a hospital setting. This is not necessarily a matter of malingering. It is more likely related to the tendency of hospitals to respond in a solicitous or kind manner to symptoms of depression or anxiety and thereby to reinforce them. Without being aware of their motivations, offenders in a hospital unit may learn to be sick in order to be reinforced. This same process, of course, has been repeatedly observed in noncriminal patients in civilian hospitals. A danger also exists that the denial of responsibility associated with acceptance of a sick role will generalize to other aspects of their behavior.

The institution or unit receiving the transferred inmate must be concerned about its own stability. It is required to be as deeply concerned with custody as the transferring institution. Even though offenders who are transferred may appear to be as severely disturbed as patients in any other hospital, they often do not stay that way. Many who are initially psychotic or severely depressed quickly reconstitute in the hospital setting and revert back to their antisocial and predatory ways. Offenders whose psychological status changes quickly from psychosis to personality disorder once they are hospitalized pose special problems for security hospitals.

The conscientious clinician must weigh a variety of complex factors in making or sanctioning the apparently simple decision to transfer an inmate from one unit to another; more factors have to be weighed than in the free world when hospitalization is at issue. Often, a wise decision in the correctional setting would seem aberrant in the free world. Inmates with minor disorders may have to be transferred to a hospital for reasons of safety, while very disturbed inmates may have to be treated in prison units because the long-term risks of transfer (such as loss of dignity and self-esteem) outweigh the short-term benefits of hospitalization.

Problems of Motivation

Irrespective of the reasons for their diversion, mentally disordered offenders are unlikely to seek treatment with enthusiasm. Some may be motivated to seek help but deny the seriousness of their difficulties, lest they be stigmatized or punished. Others are unable to comprehend their need for psychological assistance, or anticipate so little reinforcement or gratification in life if they regain their health that they may be content to remain in the illness role. Some sex offenders may find their deviant sexual behaviors so gratifying that they will not wish to give them up. Other offenders may wish to retain their symptoms in the hope they can use the sick role to avoid punishment.

Offenders who are treated to restore their competency may have mixed feelings about returning to court. Most would prefer to be tried, but some have good reasons for delaying the process and may not be highly motivated to cooperate with interventions to restore their competency. The attitudes toward treatment of those acquitted by reason of insanity will vary, depending on the statutes governing their continued commitment. Since they have recovered from whatever illness may have influenced their criminal behavior by virtue of their having been able to stand trial, it is unlikely that they will perceive themselves as in need of much treatment when they arrive at a maximum security or ordinary mental hospital.

Their motivation for change will depend in great part upon whether they perceive their participation in the treatment process as a means of obtaining an early release. In some jurisdictions, the chance of release may be significantly increased by evidence of the offender's psychological improvement. In most, however, the influence of evidence of behavioral change on release decisions is not predictable. When judges or parole boards consider release, they may be more responsive to public pressures to keep the offender restrained than to clinical reports attesting to the offender's improvement. If aware of such attitudes, insane offenders may not be highly motivated to participate in psychological interventions.

Mentally disordered sex offenders and convicted offenders residing in prison are somewhat more likely to be cooperative patients. The former group may be motivated to seek help because they perceive their deviant sexuality as repugnant and alien. This response, however, is not common. For most mentally disordered sex offenders, motivation is enhanced primarily by the possibility that successful participation in treatment will shorten the length of their incarceration. This is most likely to occur in programs where evidence of psychological change may influence release, and less likely in settings where mentally disordered sex offenders have fixed sentences.

Convicted criminals who become mentally disordered during the process of imprisonment will usually be motivated to seek relief of their acute suffering if they can do so without stigmatization or loss of power. In some prisons with sufficient mental health facilities, outreach programs have been developed to motivate prisoners to participate in group or educational programs. These programs are usually directed toward prisoners with specific problems, such as alcoholism or sexually deviant behavior. Sometimes, clinicians make themselves available to inmates at times of crisis, successfully help them to cope with their crisis, and then use the rapport gained through such intervention to encourage them to engage in more prolonged therapeutic activities. In some settings, it is possible to provide reinforcement in the form of greater privileges for those who stay in therapy and cooperate throughout the process. In a few settings, efforts have been made to foster motivation by gentle or blunt provocation or confrontation. The hope is that, once inmates experience anxiety, their motivation for treatment will increase.

In any situation where the clinician is in a position to increase privileges for inmates or to influence release decisions, the genuineness of the inmate's motivation comes into question. Since therapists who provide reinforcements also have the power to withhold them, inmates will tend to avoid disclosing negative information about themselves and will tend to emphasize their therapeutic gains. In short, a certain amount of manipulation or "conning" of the therapist will occur. The problem in such cases is one of contrived or misdirected motivation: offenders may become more committed to convincing therapists that they have made progress than they are motivated to actually change their behavior.

Clinicians can deal with this problem in a number of ways. Some, for example, are not particularly bothered by it. They view the offender's participation in the treatment process as a desirable end in itself, even if not based on a sincere effort toward self-improvement. It is assumed that offenders will be helped in spite of their motivation. Other clinicians believe that, to the extent they control the contingencies of reinforcement in the correctional setting, it is really they who are manipulating the inmates. Perhaps the majority of clinicians working in correctional settings, however, are troubled by reporting to parole boards or prison officials when they might encourage decisions to expand or limit inmate privileges or otherwise influence the timing of their release. The concern is not only with the ethical issue involved, but also with the practical issue of promoting honest communication. Those who take this issue seriously may offer to provide treatment only on the condition that no reporting will be done that could potentially help or hurt the offender. Or, they may insist that if more than one clinician is available, evaluations of therapeutic progress must be made by a clinician who is not actually conducting the treatment. This splitting of therapeutic and administrative roles has been common practice in long-term psychiatric hospitals for several decades. It is designed to facilitate honest communication between client and therapist and to help eliminate the element of manipulation from their relationship.

Modalities of Treatment

Current Resources

With few exceptions, mentally disordered offenders receive substandard treatment. At times, it is no worse than that received by patients in public mental hospitals, but it is almost never better. Many reasons for this state of affairs have been discussed previously. Whatever the causes, the lack of therapeutic commitment in this area is troubling. Over the past decade, hundreds of articles have been written about mentally disordered offenders, but only a handful (and these are usually concerned only with sex offenders) even discuss treatment. Most of the following material on this topic is based on a survey of the limited literature, visits to institutions, long telephone conversations with colleagues who work in maximum security hospitals, and my own work experiences.

It appears that all modalities of treatment are available to mentally disordered offenders. In a recent survey of institutions that treat mentally disordered offenders, more than 90 percent reported that individual treatment plans are prepared for residents and are reviewed regularly (Kerr and Roth in press). Psychotropic medication was the most universally available form of treatment, provided by 97.6 percent of the surveyed facilities. The median percentage of inmates receiving medication was 61 percent. Ninety percent of the institutions provided some form of group or individual therapy, with a median of 60 percent of inmates participating in group therapy and 34 percent in individual therapy. Behavior modification was available in 63 percent of the institutions, with a median participation rate of 27 percent. Electroconvulsive therapy was available in 19 percent of institutions but was used so infrequently that the median rate of usage was zero.

These figures actually tell us nothing about the quality of treatment, the skills possessed by those who provide it, or the diligence with which it is pursued. In this study, more than 11 percent of the responding institutions reported that psychoanalysis was available. This is an unlikely, if not impossible, finding. It suggests either a misunderstanding of what psychoanalysis is, or a mere "puffing" of the data. There is reason to suspect that the surveyed institutions define as adequate treatment many interventions that would be viewed as inferior or substandard treatment in the free world.

Biological Treatment: Antipsychotic Drugs

Neuroleptic or antipsychotic drugs are regularly used to treat mentally disordered offenders diagnosed as psychotic. The dosage levels employed tend to be lower than those used in the ordinary hospital setting for two main reasons. First, in correctional or maximum security hospital settings, the availability of adequately trained, 24-hour nursing staff is not always ensured. The use of high dosages of neuroleptics is frequently accompanied by serious side effects, which are best diagnosed and treated in a milieu where excellent medical surveillance is available. It is particularly important that changes in autonomic nervous functioning, such as postural hypotension (a sudden drop in blood pressure upon standing up), extrapyramidal nervous system functioning, such as akathisia (a sense of restlessness and need to move about constantly), or dystonia (sudden muscle contractions) be observed. This is difficult to do without nursing staff available on a 24-hour-a-day basis.

A second reason for keeping dosages of neuroleptics low is the possibly minimal need to use these agents to control undesirable behavior. In many prisons and maximum security hospitals, mentally disordered offenders are kept in cells. Sufficient structure and control are imposed on their lives to limit their opportunity to break rules, to be violent, or to engage in bizarre conduct that would be observed and labeled offensive to others. Under such conditions, neuroleptic drugs can be prescribed for the sole purpose of relieving the offender's suffering. The situation is different from that encountered on public hospital wards, where patients have the freedom to mingle with and possibly disturb others. In these settings, neuroleptic drugs tend to be used not only to alleviate suffering but also to maintain a peaceful environment. (I do not wish to imply that antipsychotic drugs are never used to control behavior in the forensic or correctional setting. This certainly happens in some institutions, and inmates complain about it bitterly. My experience has been, however, that in the better forensic institutions neuroleptics are used prudently and that they are less likely to be used for control purposes than in ordinary hospitals.)

Some of the legal issues related to the use of neuroleptic drugs in the correctional or maximum security hospital setting have been referred to previously. Inmates may not wish to receive neuroleptic medication, and most observers I have contacted agree that such refusals are usually honored in the correctional setting. Once inmates have been formally adjudicated as mentally disordered and are believed to be psychotic, however, practices tend to be different. The incompetency of psychotic inmates (usually those found incompetent to stand trial or criminally insane or those formally transferred) to consent to or refuse treatment tends to be assumed, and if treatment is refused, they are often treated on an involuntary basis. The right to refuse antipsychotic medication is protected somewhat more stringently in public hospitals, where a great deal of attention is paid to assessing the competency of committed patients. In some instances, treatment will not be imposed upon nonconsenting patients who are viewed as competent, unless an emergency arises or they are judged to be dangerous to themselves or others.

When offenders consent to pharmacological treatment in the correctional or forensic setting, they are also likely to do so with less information regarding side effects than patients in public mental hospitals. In the past decade, clinicians have become more diligent in sharing information with patients. However, some kinds of information psychiatrists do not regularly share. Provision of information regarding the side effects of tardive dyskinesia (an irreversible condition caused by prolonged use of neuroleptics and characterized by involuntary movements of the mouth, tongue, trunk, and extremities) has rarely been exhaustive in most clinical settings. It is difficult to tell highly disturbed people that drugs that are very likely to help them can also cause a disfiguring condition. Given the nature of the clients and the shortages of staff in the forensic or correctional setting, it is unlikely that much effort is devoted to providing mentally disordered offenders with information regarding tardive dyskinesia or other serious side effects of medication. It is also possible that psychiatrists in the forensic or correctional setting are less concerned about tardive dyskinesia because they see less of it. As a group, mentally disordered offenders, particularly those incompetent to stand trial and those transferred to hospitals from prison, tend to be treated for shorter periods and with lower dosages of medication than ordinary patients. Since the incidence of tardive dyskinesia is related to high dosages and prolonged treatment, the condition may be less prevalent in the correctional or forensic setting.

Antidepressant and Lithium Therapy

Antidepressant medication is available in prisons and maximum security hospitals but probably is not used frequently enough. As noted previously, depression tends to be underdiagnosed in these settings. Effective treatment with antidepressant medication requires considerable monitoring of the patients' responses and regulation of dosages. It is difficult to provide this kind of service in an understaffed custodial setting. There is also a serious danger of overdosage with these agents, since they are toxic if taken in dosages only slightly in excess of their therapeutic range. (Some antidepressants, such as the monoamine oxidase inhibitors, may become toxic if certain foods are ingested. It may not be possible to provide offenders who are given these drugs a safe diet.) Administration of antidepressive drugs to disturbed inmates must be carefully controlled. It is sometimes necessary, for example, to ascertain that inmates are not "cheeking" the drug and accumulating a sufficient number to attempt suicide.

Lithium therapy is also underused with mentally disordered offenders, probably because its use requires regular laboratory monitoring of blood levels. In some institutions, adequate laboratory facilities are not available. Underusage of lithium may also be related to limitations of the quality and quantity of staff. The willingness to diagnose bipolar affective disorders (which are usually associated with agitated or manic behavior) and to treat them with lithium is a relatively new phenomenon in American psychiatry. Psychiatrists who have not kept up with changing diagnostic and treatment trends are slow to use lithium. (It is probably used too infrequently in public hospitals, as well as in prisons and security hospitals.) All of this is unfortunate, because it is likely that a high percentage of mentally disordered offenders who are psychotic have bipolar or manic disorders. The hyperactivity, the irritability, and the grandiosity associated with mania are also likely to increase the probability of antisocial conduct. While no current studies relate bipolar affective disorders to criminal behavior, most psychiatrists who work with offenders feel that if any consistent relationship exists between psychosis and criminality, it is in this particular area.

Antianxiety Drugs

Antianxiety drugs, including barbiturates or the new benzo-diazepines such as Valium or Dalmane, are used infrequently in correctional or forensic hospital settings for several reasons. Prison or hospital staff may be reluctant to use these drugs because of punitive attitudes toward offenders. Antianxiety drugs are some-times seen as "happiness" pills which, much like alcohol or nar-cotics, could be used to diminish the painfulness of everyday prison life. When the drugs are available, they can become highly prized contraband and encourage the development of illicit marketing practices within the institution. Prison authorities are also concerned that a large number of mentally disordered of-fenders who are former drug addicts might abuse and quickly be-come addicted to any kind of agent that reduces anxiety.

In many institutions, offenders who complain of anxiety are in-correctly treated with small doses of neuroleptic medication. These agents have more serious side effects (e.g., tardive dyskinesia) than antianxiety drugs and are not really effective agents for most forms of anxiety. Indeed, they will often increase the patient's anxiety. Moreover, when it comes to the treatment of disability manifested by anxiety, mentally disordered offenders are at a dis-tinct disadvantage to other psychiatric patients. In the noncriminal population, treatment with antianxiety agents is almost routine for patients who appear to be anxious. Problems of habituation or ad-diction are usually avoided by counseling the patient and by care-fully monitoring dosages. Used in moderation during periods of high stress, these drugs are remarkably effective. They have made life less painful for many millions of citizens and have become the most frequently prescribed medications in the world. But by virtue of being prisoners, offenders are often denied a medical treatment that is available to all other citizens.

Our moralism in this area, in addition to allowing offenders to endure unnecessary pain, may well be costly to the criminal jus-tice system and society as a whole. If prisoners were allowed to use antianxiety agents (and perhaps even narcotics) freely, and if the supply of such agents were made contingent upon good behav-ior, it would be much easier to run prisons in a peaceful manner. It could be argued, however, that this is nothing but a recom-mendation for creating more drug addicts or simply a ruthless form of behavior control, although both arguments are easily rebutted. Offenders could always be withdrawn from the agent to which they are addicted shortly before their release. (Withdrawal from either benzodiazepines or narcotics is not nearly as difficult a problem as most persons believe.) The behavior control argument can be countered by pointing out that drugs need never be forced upon inmates. They might simply be made available as one more reinforcer, similar to such privileges as watching television. As compared with other methods currently used to control criminal behavior, the contingent use of psychotropic drugs would be far from the cruelest.

Restricting the use of antianxiety drugs in the criminal justice system has other adverse consequences. As in the free world, the banning of any medication that alleviates pain helps to create a new and illicit industry, namely, drug trafficking. Antianxiety drugs (as well as stimulants and narcotics) are available on an illegal basis in almost all jails and many prisons. They are also available, to a lesser extent, in security hospitals. Ironically, our moralism leads to corruption of prison workers and the family members of offenders, who ultimately are the most likely persons to smuggle these agents into institutions. The presence of illicit drugs in custodial settings also encourages occasional mortal battles among inmates seeking to gain power within the institution. Most disturbing, illicit drugs become a powerful reinforcer that is controlled entirely by the inmate subculture rather than by institutional officials.

Electroconvulsive Therapy

Another biological intervention that is rarely used in the correctional or forensic setting is electroconvulsive therapy (ECT). Convincing evidence shows that ECT is a highly effective treatment for severe depression, schizophrenia, and maniaoconditions not uncommon among offenders. Unfortunately, ECT has gained a reputation for being a highly intrusive and permanently mind-altering intervention. Although this reputation is undeserved, the courts and legislatures have been persuaded to require a number of procedural precautions before it can be used. And, it is especially difficult these days to give ECT to nonconsenting patients. In most states, even civilly committed patients cannot be given ECT without their consent, unless they are found incompetent and court-appointed guardians agree to the treatment. Private hospitals with sufficient staff to take the time to go through the legal processes necessary to use this treatment on reluctant patients still use ECT frequently. Public hospitals, on the other hand, are rapidly abandoning its use. Ironically, ECT, which was once viewed as an intervention imposed primarily upon poor and helpless involuntary patients is now available primarily to the affluent.

Even if patients consent to receive ECT, many public and security hospitals do not have a sufficient number of staff members willing or able to provide the treatment. More and more public hospitals are simply sending their patients to community or university hospitals when they need ECT. Only an occasional security hospital has sufficient personnel or facilities for administering this treatment. All of this is discouraging, since a preponderance of evidence indicates that ECT in its modern form of administration is a safe and highly effective treatment for many of the disorders plaguing offenders. (My views here are certainly biased by past experience. I began working in hospitals for the criminally insane 30 years ago, before neuroleptic medication was readily available or was considered the preferred treatment for psychosis. In those days, ECT was the best and usually the only treatment available. I gave ECT to hundreds of patients and, although my memory may distort, I found it was often as efficacious as current drug therapy.)

Antiandrogen Drugs

The biological treatments discussed thus far are not ordinarily used to rehabilitate but are used with the intention of alleviating disease processes that may be unrelated to the offender's criminal behavior. The only exception might involve biological treatment of insanity acquittees whose crimes are presumed to be directly related to their illnesses. Mentally disordered sex offenders, however, are sometimes treated with very powerful biological interventions for the direct purpose of rehabilitation. In Europe, castration has been used for over a decade as a treatment for recidivistic sex offenders (Sturup 1972). Some researchers have reported excellent results with this procedure, but its true efficacy and its ethical propriety are still subjects of debate. In the United States during the past decade, various drugs that reduce sexual drive have been used on a voluntary basis. These drugs, called antiandrogens, have the advantage of not producing permanent castration. When they are discontinued, the offender's sexual capacities return. The most frequently used agent is cyproterone acetate, which lowers the level of circulating male hormone in the bloodstream. This drug can be injected in long-acting "depo" form so that it does not have to be given on a frequent basis.

Antiandrogens are given only to offenders who consent to their use. (While offenders must volunteer for this treatment, substantial coercion may still be involved in its use: offenders may be given the choice of taking the drugs or serving a long prison sentence.) The "depo" form of cyproterone acetate (called depo provera) is used to maintain androgen levels at a low level for months at a time. In this condition of "chemical castration," the offender's sexual urges and sexual capacities are substantially diminished. As a rule, offenders who are receiving this drug stop all sexual activity. Antiandrogens appear to have an especially favorable effect on sex offenders who have abnormally high sex drives and who are plagued with fantasies of deviant sexual activity on a day-to-day or even hour-to-hour basis (Walker and Meyer 1981). During the course of antiandrogen therapy, these patients experience a sense of relief from the pressure of sexual impluses. They are reported to be especially amenable to conventional therapy during this period of artificially induced sexual quiescence. Even after the treatment is stopped, some subjects report that their sexual drive is much more manageable and can be channeled in non-deviant directions (Perkins 1983). Treatment with antiandrogens may be especially helpful to older sex offenders who have little opportunity or ability to develop socially acceptable alternatives to deviant sexuality. Faced with a choice of either continuing deviant activity with the associated risk of frequent imprisonment or giving up sexuality altogether, they may elect the latter.

If antiandrogen therapy should continue to prove efficacious, a new commitment could be seen in the criminal justice system to using biological interventions to rehabilitate criminals. Expanded use of such agents, however, will raise substantial ethical and legal questions regarding such issues as voluntariness of consent and "mind control." A little over a decade ago, for example, a Michigan court ruled that an involuntarily committed sex offender could not consent to experimental psychosurgery (*Kaimowitz v. Department of Mental Health* 1973). The court ruled that a patient committed to a correctional institution could not give a voluntary, informed, and competent consent to a treatment so intrusive and permanent in its effects as psychosurgery. It also noted that such treatment could infringe on the first amendment right to "generate ideas" as well as the right to privacy. While reversible "chemical castration" may not be as intrusive or permanent as psychosurgery, its use, especially as an alternative to imprisonment, raises similar legal issues. Thus far, no legal challenges to the use of depo provera have been raised, but since it appears that it is being widely used in correctional and security hospital settings, it should not be surprising if current practices are soon challenged in the courts.

Behavior Modification for Rehabilitation or Adjustment Purposes

Behavior therapy has an uncertain role in the correctional and forensic setting. Many of the original behavior modification efforts consisted of involuntary programs for mentally disordered offenders that were designed to control their behavior within institutions. It was also hoped that such behavioral change would influence the offenders' subsequent behavior upon release and would, therefore, be rehabilitative. Most of these programs were poorly conceptualized from both a scientific and a humanitarian standpoint. The most controversial involved the use of aversive conditioning. In one institution, apomorphine, which induces severe nausea and vomiting, was administered by nonphysicians to nonconsenting offenders as a part of an aversive conditioning program (*Knecht v. Gillman* 1973). When prisoners misbehaved, they were simply given the drug with the intent of producing painful consequences to discourage antisocial conduct. In another institution, succinylcholine, which temporarily paralyzes the muscles (including those that control breathing), was administered to inmates who had done something prohibited. This drug induces feelings of extreme fear and helplessness. While in this state of anguish, subjects were given lectures on the wrongfulness of their behavior (*Mackey v. Procunier* 1973). Both of these programs resulted in litigation, in which the courts concluded that the administration of such substances, without patient consent, amounted to cruel and unusual punishment and should be prohibited.

Other programs based on principles of operant conditioning also paid little attention to offenders' rights and were quickly abandoned because of court restraining orders or fear of litigation. These programs were based on the assumption that certain offenders who had severe adjustment problems within institutions could benefit by being deprived of most of the reinforcers they enjoyed in daily life (comfortable clothes, a comfortable bed, decent food, interpersonal contact, reading material, tobacco, recreation) and then gradually having these reinforcers restored, contingent upon good behavior (Wexler 1973). The principle here is similar to that involved in creating token economies or in treating such disorders as anorexia nervosa. In the case of prisoners, however, the "privileges" that were taken away so that they could earn them back through good behavior were basic amenities of a decent existence. The involuntary nature of these programs, coupled with the extreme deprivation they imposed upon offenders, quickly led to litigation that encouraged their abandonment.

Because of their controversial nature, it is unlikely that extensive programs of behavior modification have been implemented and sustained in American prisons and forensic hospitals for periods longer than a few months. Little likelihood exists that this situation will soon change. The terms "behavior therapy" or "behavior modification" still evoke suspicion and concern on the part of those concerned with the rights of offenders. When behavior modification programs are proposed in correctional or forensic settings, a predictable protest arises from many libertarian groups along with a corollary probability that litigation will be initiated to stop them. Currently, the Federal Bureau of Prisons is so concerned with such protest and litigation that it will not even support research on behavior modification in its institutions.

With all of society's fears and antagonisms toward behavior modification, it is important to recognize that principles of learning or conditioning are always operating upon offenders. Any time an institution takes control of a person's life and regulates most of the reinforcements and punishments the person can experience, it is exerting a powerful form of behavior modification. While we do not usually think of the day-to-day regulation of prison behavior as behavior therapy, the only difference between this form of regulating behavior and the regulation resulting from "real" behavior therapy is that, in the latter, the contingencies of reinforcement or punishment are spelled out with more precision. The day-to-day behavior modification that goes on in our correctional institutions and forensic hospitals tends to be sloppy, inconsistent, and unscientific. Much greater emphasis is placed on punishment than on reinforcement. Inmates learn that they will be punished *unless* they engage in certain behaviors (negative reinforcement) or because they indulge in prohibited behaviors. They are rarely reinforced for engaging in socially acceptable behaviors; they simply lose reinforcement when they do not. In this situation, they fail to learn alternative and acceptable behaviors. Most learning theorists would argue that learning proceeds most effectively when positive reinforcement and the possibility of learning alternative behavior are emphasized, rather than punishment. Nevertheless, this is exactly the opposite of how we currently use behavior modification in our correctional and forensic institutions.

While the behavior modification programs that have been litigated out of existence probably deserved their fate, the criminal justice system's rejection of such programs is not entirely rational. It would not be too difficult to devise programs based on a consistent use of reinforcement that would not infringe on the rights of offenders and that might be effective in influencing at least their behavior within the institution. Such programs might appropriately be viewed simply as efforts to systematize and humanize the crude forms of behavior modification that naturally occur within institutions. Even if aversive consequences were to be used as part of a behavior modification program, the punishments imposed upon offenders need not be any more cruel than those that are currently viewed as acceptable punishment in correctional institutions.

Behavior Therapy: Less Controversial Uses

Less controversial forms of behavior therapy that do not raise too many legal or ethical questions are used in correctional and forensic settings to alleviate the suffering of selected mentally disordered offenders. Offenders who respond to certain benign environmental stimuli with intense and unrealistic fear, and who are diagnosed as having phobic disorders, can be treated by exposure to the feared stimulus using various techniques, such as systematic desensitization and flooding (Emmelkamp 1982). So can offenders who have compulsions based on avoidance of feared stimuli. The principle involved in all of these interventions is that of placing the patient in the feared situation under circumstances in which no aversive consequences will follow. (In systematic desensitization, exposure is gradual and painless; in flooding, exposure is massive and highly stressful.) If repeated exposure is not followed by aversive events, the phobic response is likely to be extinguished. One problem with using this kind of treatment in the prison or forensic setting is that it is often difficult to determine whether the offender's fear of certain stimuli is actually unrealistic. A fear of going out in the prison "yard" is not unrealistic when the risks of assault in that setting are great. Viewing this fear as a phobia and treating it as such may not be in the best interest of the offender.

In dealing with generalized anxiety, offenders can benefit from learning some form of the relaxation response, either through deep muscular relaxation, autogenic therapy, imagery, hypnosis, or transcendental meditation (biofeedback technology usually not being available) (Benson et al. 1974). Selected offenders receive this type of training when clinicians (usually psychologists) are available to offer it. In most institutions, these techniques are not available.

Role modeling and behavioral rehearsal may be used to help offenders deal either with personal problems or with the ultimate goal of moving forward in the justice process. Some incompetent defendants attend classes where they learn about the criminal trial and how they can cooperate with attorneys and assist in their own defense. A mock court trial can be set up, with other inmates playing the roles of the various participants, and each inmate can rehearse the role of being a defendant in court. The class leader can also model competent behavior in the various situations defendants might encounter. As a rule, assertiveness training is not encouraged in correctional or forensic settings (usually because of the fear that it will make inmates less cooperative and more belligerent). However, inmates in protective custody settings, who tend to be frequently exploited by other inmates, are sometimes taught nonviolent ways of protecting themselves. Role modeling and behavioral rehearsal may be used in this process.

Other types of social skills training are sometimes available for sex offenders and are used with the ultimate goal of rehabilitation. A certain number of sex offenders lack the kind of skills that might enable them to meet, converse with, and become intimate with mature partners of the opposite sex. If they can learn these skills through role modeling and behavioral rehearsal, it is hoped they will have enhanced motivations to seek socially acceptable sexual interactions. The degree of efficacy of these techniques is, of course, limited by the availability of females who can work with offenders and the limits that must be placed on their interaction with offenders. Some clinicians have postulated that certain sex deviants may simply be frightened of relating to mature heterosexual partners. If the specific feared stimuli related to social encounters with females can be identified, a variety of techniques useful in treating phobias may be equally helpful.

Other behavioral techniques alleged to rehabilitate sex offenders and not pose an overwhelming ethical issue are covert sensitization and shaping. In covert sensitization, subjects are taught to pair an unpleasant thought with a fantasy of their preferred deviant sexual activity. Since the aversive stimulus is only a thought or image suggested by the therapist, rather than an action (such as electric shock), this treatment is not viewed as intrusive or cruel. With shaping techniques, offenders are encouraged to gradually change their sexual fantasies so they can be directed toward appropriate activities (lovemaking rather than rape) or appropriate objects (adults rather than children). In outpatient settings, practice with adult sexual surrogates, both homosexual and heterosexual, is possible. The goal is to gradually shape the individual's preferences toward mature rather than immature partners (McConaghy 1982).

The techniques of covert sensitization and shaping can be assisted by new developments in measuring penile tumescence. Sex offenders may show more erectile response to deviant than to socially acceptable sexual stimuli (Abel et al. 1977). The capacity to measure the offender's erectile response to various auditory and visual stimuli gives clinicians a relatively objective criterion for assessing their improvement. It must be noted, however, that subjects often have some control of their erectile responses and may consciously inhibit a response to a deviant stimulus in order to impress the therapist.

A more ethically questionable form of behavior therapy involves the association of a mild aversive stimulus (chemically induced nausea, unpleasant smells, mild electric shocks to the arm) with a deviant sexual stimulus (presented via slides, films, or audiotapes). The aversive stimulus may be paired with the deviant stimulus (classical conditioning), may follow it (operant conditioning), or may be avoided if the offender elects to turn off the deviant stimulus (anticipatory avoidance conditioning) (Marks et al. 1970). Sometimes these techniques are followed by aversive relief, a procedure that pairs the cessation of an aversive stimulus with the appearance of a socially acceptable sexual stimulus. A picture of a nude adult of the opposite sex may, for example, be flashed on a screen just as a painful shock is stopped. The patient presumably comes to associate the heterosexual stimulus with the relieved state that follows the cessation of pain or discomfort.

I have listed a number of behavioral techniques that can be used to treat mentally disordered offenders. The reader should not assume that all of these techniques have been proven useful or that they are readily available to offenders. Most of the techniques of behavior modification designed to rehabilitate sex offenders are best viewed as experimental. They have been tried on only small numbers of subjects and with inconsistent results. It is also difficult to find skilled behavior therapists in correctional or forensic settings. In reality, only a small number of mentally disordered offenders receive any form of scientifically based behavior therapy.

Psychotherapy

Determining how much psychotherapy is available to mentally disordered offenders is difficult, as much disagreement exists as to which verbal interactions between institution staff and inmates should be called psychotherapy and which are guidance or counseling. A certain number of people in the prison or forensic hospital, including correctional officers and ministers, are always willing to listen empathically to the offender's problem and maybe offer advice. Whether or not such interventions constitute psychotherapy, they are often very helpful to the inmate. Formal individual psychotherapy (defined as a treatment in which a trained person deliberately establishes a professional relationship with an emotionally troubled person and, through a process of mostly verbal interaction, helps the troubled person find a more comfortable and effective adaptation) is available to only a few inmates. The primary reason for this is the scarcity of trained professionals in prisons and forensic hospitals. Psychotherapy takes up a good deal of the therapist's time and is usually viewed as the least cost-effective intervention. Criminologists also have a widespread belief that, while psychotherapy may help those offenders with mental disorders to feel better and to function more effectively within institutions, it will have no impact on their subsequent criminality. States have been reluctant to support expensive psychotherapy programs that promise only to restore to health and do not hold out the promise of rehabilitation.

The situation with regard to sex offenders is somewhat different. In dealing with this group, some belief prevails that psychotherapy can modify their motivations to commit deviant sexual acts and can help them learn to find alternative and socially acceptable sources of sexual gratification. Psychotherapy for these persons is viewed as rehabilitative. Currently, a few psychotherapists are available to work with sex offenders, both in indeterminate programs and in ordinary correctional settings.

The techniques used to treat sex offenders vary from psychoanalytic and Rogerian to confrontational and exhortative. The skills of the therapists vary from exceptional to poor. Some highly skilled and dedicated but unheralded therapists have worked for years in prison or hospital settings providing intensive psychotherapy to sex offenders. They do some followup studies of their patients and insist their interventions are quite helpful (Groth 1979). The difficulties in evaluating the legitimacy of claims that psychotherapy helps sex offenders are, of course, legion. Psychotherapy is a difficult intervention to evaluate in any setting. The problems in evaluating its efficiency with offenders are even greater, and it is especially difficult to evaluate treatment results. The failure of offenders to recidivate may be viewed as a criterion of success, but it may be impossible to determine whether they have truly abandoned antisocial behavior patterns or if various other factors, including improved skill in avoiding arrest, have enabled them to avoid conviction.

Carefully controlled studies of the efficacy of treating sex offenders are, for practical purposes, nonexistent. Legal and moral problems are involved in defining some persons as extremely dangerous and then designating them part of a control group that will not be treated. Legislators are naturally reluctant to draft statutes that allow for the differential treatment of dangerous offenders who have committed the same crimes, and clinicians are reluctant to withhold treatments they believe are beneficial from control groups. (It may be appropriate to note here that while no scientific evidence proves that psychotherapy rehabilitates offenders, there certainly is no proof that it does not. A high recidivism rate following psychotherapy can be blamed on deficiencies in the type of therapy or the skill of therapists, on the difficulty of doing psychotherapy in the repressive milieu of the prison, or on the inordinate stress society imposes upon offenders who have been released.)

Group therapy is more common than individual psychotherapy in correctional and forensic settings. Here again, however, a definitional problem occurs. In some correctional settings staff members, including correctional officers who have very little training, assume the responsibility of meeting regularly with inmate groups. While they may use some of the principles of psychotherapy in their work, they can hardly be viewed as skilled professionals. The focus of this kind of group work tends to be on controlling the behavior of offenders within the institution. In contrast, professional clinicians are more likely to do group psychotherapy with the goal of rehabilitation.

Some clinicians believe that sex offenders are more likely to be rehabilitated by participating in group than in individual psychotherapy. Presumably, in group therapy sex offenders will discover that others in the "same boat" will understand them; this understanding should, in theory, be emotionally supportive and should enhance their willingness to cooperate by freely disclosing their problems. Groups designed to rehabilitate offenders use a variety of techniques. Some are primarily educational. The leaders show films and give lectures that clarify the nature of emotional problems. Other groups rely on exhortation or principles of behavior modification. Most commonly, groups in correctional or forensic settings rely heavily on interaction between members. The leader confronts the group members and urges them to confront one another. The leader will also stress the need for offenders to acknowledge responsibility for their behavior (Green 1984).

It is extremely difficult to do family therapy in prisons or maximum security hospitals. Geographic variables may impose insurmountable handicaps. Most families of mentally disordered offenders cannot afford to make trips to remote institutions with any regularity. Some family members may be reluctant to visit the treatment site, and children, who may be critical participants in the treatment process, may not be allowed to visit. The prisoner's diminished status with regard to the rest of the family may also adversely influence therapeutic outcome. Family therapists prefer to work in a setting where the "identified" patient is not viewed as more disturbed or disadvantaged than any other family member (Whitaker 1978). Obviously, the fact of imprisonment puts the mentally disordered offender in a severely compromised position relative to the rest of the family. Under these conditions, it is easy for family members to impute blame to the patient without looking at their own roles in influencing the offender's behavior.

Offenders are in an especially vulnerable position when expressing any negative feelings toward family members. In the course of family therapy, it is almost always useful for such feelings to be at least shared. But incarcerated offenders must be concerned that, if they express too many negative feelings toward loved ones, they may simply refuse to return for further therapy or even for further visits. Finally, family members do not have the opportunity to go off and work things out together after the therapeutic hour as they do in the free world. A moment of un-

derstanding cannot be fully enjoyed; a moment of tension cannot
be worked through.

Problems in Providing Psychotherapy

Certain problems are inherent in providing effective psychotherapy of any type in the correctional or forensic setting. I have
already noted that offenders may be less motivated to change their
behavior than other clients and will be unlikely to present their
problems honestly in situations where their therapists can influence the privileges they receive or their release date. However,
several other problems peculiar to prisons and security hospitals
complicate the task of therapy. Five such dilemmas are discussed
here.

1. *Clinicians cannot be assured that clients will appear at a
scheduled therapy session.* Prisons and forensic hospitals are administered by individuals whose first concern must be security.
Inmates who are being punished or who are felt to be at risk of
being disruptive may not be allowed to attend therapy sessions.
Also, other institutional needs must occasionally take precedence
over therapy. The hours during which inmates can work, play, eat,
sleep, and have visitors are strictly regulated, so it may be very
difficult to schedule or reschedule a therapy session. If the institutional routine is for any reason disrupted, the therapy hour may
be the first event canceled.

2. *Confidentiality is a special problem in treating mentally disordered offenders.* In the free world, confidentiality is an essential
aspect of successful psychotherapy. Confidential material is not
usually shared with third parties unless patients request it or unusual circumstances arise. In working with mentally disordered offenders, therapists are often encouraged to share their patients'
disclosures with other members of the prison or hospital staff. At
times, however, such sharing can become a formidable impedi-
ment to developing an honest therapeutic relationship. Nevertheless, some information revealed in therapy must be shared with
other members of the prison or hospital staff. Anything the inmate
might reveal that threatens the integrity of the institution cannot
be viewed as privileged information. Also, confidentiality is impossible when inmates announce plans to escape or to harm others.
The situation is more equivocal when patients tell therapists about
the potential antisocial behavior of other inmates. In these situations, therapists must consider the possibility that their clients'

perceptions are inaccurate. The advantages of sharing their clients' communications must be weighed against the problems that disclosure might create for the inmate, the institution, or the therapeutic relationship.

3. *The correctional or forensic setting presents a paucity of experiences to complement and validate the learning that goes on in psychotherapy.* Offenders cannot generalize their learning in psychotherapy to real-life situations. (This problem of lack of generalization occurs with behavior therapy as well as with psychotherapy.) For example, individuals may learn to be assertive in therapy but have no opportunity to experiment with assertiveness within the institution. Inmates may develop powerful insights into the roots of problems, such as sexual deviation, but have no opportunity to experiment with alternative behaviors. Nor can inmates test out how they would respond to the stresses they will encounter in the free world. Prisons are stressful, but they do not necessarily impose the same kind of stresses that may have elicited the offender's antisocial behavior. Although offenders may seem to be "cured" in a custodial setting, neither they nor their therapists can be assured that treatment has really worked. The artificiality of psychotherapy in a rigidly controlled institutional setting may have a great deal to do with its limited value as a rehabilitative technique.

4. *Therapists who work with offenders have little power to make recommendations that lead to changes in environmental situations conducive to their patients' mental health.* Changes in working or sleeping arrangements, or in the availability of recreational activities, may make an important difference in the patient's adjustment. A simple example of this would be the recommendation commonly made in mental health practice that an anxious patient take up an exercise program, such as jogging on a regular basis. Such a recommendation might be very difficult to implement in an institutional setting, however. Issues such as institutional needs and the policies of trying to treat all inmates exactly the same make it difficult to tailor any type of milieu program to the needs of a particular client.

5. *The nature of what is sometimes called transference and countertransference is distorted in institutional settings.* Many of the attitudes and responses offenders develop toward therapists are deleterious to the therapeutic process. Some of these attitudes and responses may not be related to the offender's past learning but rather are determined by the institutional setting. Qualities such as dependency and passive aggressiveness toward authority figures

are quickly learned in prison and security hospitals. Thus, if offenders relate to therapists in these ways, it is extremely difficult to determine how much of their response should be interpreted as transference, based on distorted past learning experiences, and how much accepted as realistic and adaptive.

Therapists have a different set of problems. Mentally disordered offenders are often highly disturbed people who are likely to bring a great deal of aggressive and sexual material into the therapy hour. This material might be difficult for some therapists to deal with in any setting. In a custodial setting where tensions are high, where impulses are strong, and where the possible responses to deviation are so punitive, therapists may experience dealing with such material as highly stressful. This is more than what is usually called countertransference. It is extremely hard to avoid developing deep feelings toward those who are undergoing the ordeal of involuntary confinement, and empathic therapists will invariably experience some of the pain that afflicts their clients.

Treatment in the Community

Up to now, I have considered treatment of institutionalized offenders only. In the community, once again, mentally disordered offenders tend to receive substandard treatment. Community mental health centers are usually reluctant to work with them. Few offenders can afford the luxury of a private therapist. In many jurisdictions, it is unclear which social service agency will be responsible for their outpatient supervision and treatment. Prerelease counseling tends to be limited in most institutions, and little liaison exists between security hospitals and community agencies. Once in the community, mentally disordered offenders encounter all of the problems of exprisoners on parole, but with the additional handicaps of dealing with a possibly still-unresolved mental illness and the stigma resulting from being labeled mentally ill.

The major community programs available for noninstitutionalized mentally disordered offenders are directed toward those who have committed minor offenses that the community does not feel warrant prolonged restraint. Some court-attached social agencies have worked in conjunction with mental health centers to provide a full range of services to help sustain these persons in the community (Brodsky 1982). They may provide medication and psychotherapy as well as the usual social services. Efforts are made to keep offenders gainfully occupied or, at the very least, to provide them with food and shelter. In times of stress, treatment emphasis is placed on making counselors who use techniques of crisis intervention readily available to help their clients develop socially acceptable responses. These community treatment services are helpful to both offenders and society. They are vcertainly preferable alternatives to jailing minor offenders who are mentally disordered, or to "shipping" them off to remote security hospitals to have their competency evaluated.

CHAPTER 8

Ethical Issues

EFFORTS TO DEAL WITH mentally disordered offenders create formidable ethical problems for clinicians and for society. Some of these same problems also arise in dealing with civil patients. However, where punishment is a possible outcome of clinical or societal practices, the ethical conflicts are more powerful.

Double Agent Roles

The most troubling problem for clinicians who work in the criminal justice system is that their diagnostic and therapeutic skills enable them to obtain information from offenders that, once communicated to judicial agencies, can lead to dispositions offenders would not welcome. A clinical evaluation, for example, may influence decisions to place offenders in prison. It may be relied upon to determine the length of their sentences, or it may be a critical factor in influencing the judge or jury to impose the death penalty. Psychiatric evaluation may also be influential in determining whether offenders will continue to be incarcerated or will be released.

The ethical issue is most troubling when the clinician is hired by the prosecution or is state-employed. In these situations, offenders may experience unwelcome consequences as a result of an evaluation they have not sought. They may not wish to be found incompetent or insane, or they may be wary of the consequences of transfer from a prison to a hospital. They will certainly not welcome the consequences of being labeled dangerous. The ethical issues are less critical, however, when clinicians are employed by defendants. Under these circumstances, it is probable that the clinicians' recommendations will be congruent with the wishes of offenders. But even when they hire their own experts, offenders sustain some risk. Many forensic experts, irrespective of who employs them, feel ethically obligated to include in their reports material that may reflect adversely upon their clients. In some jurisdictions, the material may become available to the prosecution or state agencies and may be used to justify dispositions offenders may not welcome.

When clinicians are in a position to do things their patients may experience as harmful, they assume a rather unusual role. In the mind of the public, clinicians, and especially doctors, have no professional commitments other than those they owe to their patients. Most people view a doctor or psychotherapist as somebody whose only obligation is to help people. While offenders may be cynical and suspicious of authority figures, they too have been trained to trust doctors. When a doctor asks them questions, they, like all other citizens, have been "programmed" to try to respond truthfully. But telling the truth to a state- or prosecution-employed expert may hurt the offender. This is a confusing situation for offenders, who cannot determine if the evaluator is their friend or their adversary. Since evaluators in these circumstances have dual allegiances, partly to the offender and perhaps more to the agency that employs them, they are sometimes described as working in a "double agent" role (Szasz 1963).

Clinicians may contribute to the ambiguity of their role when they themselves are confused and ambivalent about their obligations. On the one hand, clinicians who are employed by the state or prosecution are aware that they have certain commitments to society. On the other hand, by virtue of having committed themselves to careers as helping persons, they also want to help their patients. Often, they do not wish to acknowledge their dual allegiances or their "double agent" roles, either to themselves or to their clients. In conducting interviews with offenders, even state-employed clinicians are likely to use the same kinds of skills and techniques they would employ in the evaluation of any other patient. Most of these technical maneuvers convey to offenders that they are in the presence of a helping person. Offenders in this situation may have limited awareness that their evaluators can make recommendations for dispositions that will hurt them.

One important technique psychiatrists and other evaluators use to gain rapport with and encourage communication from offenders is showing empathy or a compassionate understanding of their emotional state. Another technique requires the selective use of reinforcement, either by words, gesture, or facial expression, to keep their clients talking about relevant issues. It is almost impossible for clinicians, whatever their function, to avoid using this technique as well as others such as clarification and interpretation. Clinicians seek maximum information. Patients communicate best when they feel liked and understood. Because clinicians must use all of their technical skills to conduct an adequate evaluation, offenders are at risk of believing they are in a therapeutic encounter. They may, in effect, be seduced into revealing information that could be used against them.

The problem has both legal and ethical ramifications. Various legal authorities have proposed that offenders should have attorneys present at the time of their evaluation to instruct them as to which questions should be answered (Ennis and Embry 1978). This proposal would effectively eliminate the possibility of accurate evaluation and, it is hoped, will not be taken seriously by our legislators or courts. A more practical manner of dealing with this problem has been proposed by the American Psychiatric Association's Task Force on the Role of Psychiatry in the Sentencing Process (Halleck 1984). In looking at the psychiatrist's shifting allegiances to the individual and the state, this report first seeks to develop a value system for approaching the problem. The report (American Psychiatric Association 1984) notes:

> Even those who advocate a primary devotion to judicial needs are unlikely to ignore the manifest needs of the individual who is currently the focus of their attention. No ethical psychiatrist examining defendants for a court would permit obvious and previously unrecognized psychiatric illness to go unmentioned because of its irrelevance to the determination at hand. On the other hand, even the most individually oriented psychiatrist is faced with the need to compromise that orientation to meet certain broader needs, for example, the protection of society. Psychiatrists are required by law to report child abuse. They participate in civil commitment proceedings which are designed to protect the public from "dangerous" patients. They appreciate their obligation to try to prevent their patients from committing violent acts.
>
> Since some compromise between these two extremes is inevitable, the only question is at what point to strike the balance. We recognize that one legal value must be given primacy in presentencing evaluations—the need to determine the truth. Agreeing to participate in the sentencing process therefore obligates the psychiatrist to make a good faith effort to conduct a

thorough examination. It also precludes withholding any relevant information. Having thereby satisfied the obligation to society, however, the remainder of the psychiatrist's behavior should adhere to an individual-centered orientation. (pp. 192-193, reprinted with permission)

The above-stated ethical principle necessitates a firm commitment on the part of clinicians to be sure that offenders do not mistake the nature and purpose of the assessment. Using this principle, the APA task force report concludes that the offender must be provided with as much information as possible concerning the nature and purpose of the examination. Such information should include an explanation that the clinician is not functioning in a traditional medical role, but rather is serving as an agent of the court (or of the prosecution) for the purpose of gathering data that may be relevant to the determination of incompetency, insanity, or the length and nature of a criminal sentence. The circumstances under which information divulged during the evaluation may be disclosed to the prosecution or the court should be made explicit. Finally, clinicians should explain as best they can how defendants may be helped or harmed by the information in the report. This may include a brief description of the applicable law. If subjects are unclear about any of this, and matters are not clarified after they have been given an opportunity to ask questions, all examinations should be postponed until offenders have had a chance to discuss the matter with their attorneys. When it appears that defendants are incompetent to give informed consent, the clinician who wishes to conform to the APA's ethical code should stop the examination, inform the party who requested the evaluation of the defendant's condition, and allow the legal system to arrive at a solution to the problem.

Scrupulous attention to obtaining informed consent to an evaluation interview does not eliminate the possibility that defendants will reveal embarrassing material or information that may later affect them adversely. Such a risk is always present in this type of evaluation. However, it is a risk that competent offenders must assume once they are thrust into the criminal justice process.

The APA task force report also has some advice as to the stance psychiatrists should take toward using empathic and other techniques, such as clarification and interpretation, that may lower the offender's usual defenses. It concludes that these techniques must be used, not only because they represent the essence of the psychiatric examination, but because they may well be necessary to prevent offenders from suffering harm as a result of discussing psychologically distressing topics. The most that the task force advises here is that the psychiatrist should stop the examination whenever it appears the offender is confused about the purpose of the encounter. An offender who appears to be slipping into a "therapeutic" mind set should be reminded of the nontherapeutic intent of the assessment before the examination proceeds further.

General Ethical Issues

Assuming that clinicians view their function in evaluating offenders as providing society with as much truthful information as possible, an ethical as well as practical question arises as to whether this goal is most aptly fulfilled if they function as "neutral" examiners who are agents of the court, or if they should involve themselves in the adversary process as experts for the defense or prosecution. In practice, most evaluations relating to mentally disordered offenders are performed by clinicians who are state-employed and who are, in theory, neutral. Unfortunately, a strong tendency is seen for state-employed evaluators to identify more powerfully with the needs of society than with the needs of offenders. The reasons for this are not entirely clear, except that the state pays their salary and formidable pressures will be put upon them should they make recommendations resulting in harm to society. Another problem with "neutral" evaluators is that they are often the only evaluators. If their biases should happen to influence their reports, the courts will have no access to what may be more reliable and expert information.

On the other hand, some advantages go with using "neutral" evaluators. The most important of these is that they are unlikely to be pressured by conscious or unconscious motivations to "win" an adversarial proceeding at all costs. It has been my experience that psychiatrists who work for either the prosecution or the defense tend to get caught up in the adversarial process and become deeply concerned with winning or losing the case. Such concerns are perfectly appropriate for attorneys. However, too much commitment to the outcome of a legal case may encourage experts to exaggerate the strength of their own arguments and to ignore the strength of opposing arguments. Their dispassionate search for truth may be compromised and the reliability of their testimony diminished.

It is not possible to say whether neutral or adversarial testimony is most useful to the court, or which form poses the fewest ethical conflicts for mental health professionals. Neutral evaluators must guard against becoming too society-oriented and must strive for a certain degree of humility in communicating how certain they are of their findings. Experts who work for the defense or prosecution must be aware of their tendency to become advocates and must guard against allowing their commitment to a particular judicial outcome to compromise their obligation to the truth.

A final comment must be made on the morality of any member of a helping profession working in a system that deliberately inflicts pain upon its clients. Certainly, clinicians have a moral obligation to use their skills to help protect society. Clinicians have assumed social control functions in our society for many decades, and good reason exists to believe they will continue to do so. But the use of clinical skills to control the behavior of selected individuals becomes less and less justifiable when the punitive actions society takes against this group are irrational and excessive. It is my belief that the criminal justice system inflicts punishments upon offenders that are excessively cruel, often arbitrary, and usually in excess of the degree required to protect the public. If I am right, then anyone who works in such a system and *contributes* to its smooth functioning, without trying to change it or without at least acknowledging its inadequacies, becomes an apologist for an oppressive status quo (Halleck 1971). This is a troubling ethical problem for any healer. A certain amount of good can be done for society and for some individuals by participating in the various dispositional and treatment decisions about mentally disordered offenders. But to the extent that such participation is viewed or actually functions as a means of stabilizing an oppressive system, it may not be morally justifiable.

The Ethics of Rehabilitation

Current Practices

In Chapter 7, I noted that techniques originally designed to treat mental disorders could also be used to change the antisocial behavior of some offenders, even if the interventions did not alleviate a mental disorder. The goal of treatment or intervention would then be viewed as "rehabilitation only." Ordinarily, medical or behavioral technology is not used to change human behavior unless the behavior to be influenced is related to some type of recognized disorder. This is almost always the case when patients are treated under a medical model. Even the criminal justice system is wary of intervening when no documented illness is present. It permits some "rehabilitation only" interventions but restricts the use of most of them.

Currently, most correctional and forensic institutions approve of group, individual, or family psychotherapy as a rehabilitative tool, even when it is not clear that the use of this intervention is directed at a specific disorder. Psychotherapy is most likely to be approved if participation is voluntary. In a few settings, however, offenders have been compelled to attend counseling sessions that have rehabilitative goals only. This practice has aroused little protest, perhaps because psychotherapy is not viewed as a very intrusive intervention. It is often assumed that offenders can resist its effects if they really want to.

Psychotherapy is the only intervention that goes unquestioned when used for rehabilitative purposes only. Psychosurgery for even consenting mentally disordered offenders is, for all practical purposes, prohibited. Drugs of any type tend to be used for rehabilitative purposes, primarily in those few instances when it is felt they also will treat some underlying disorder. (A possible exception may be the use of long-acting antiandrogens.) Behavior modification programs receive special scrutiny by the public and the courts. Electroconvulsive treatment as a "rehabilitation only" intervention is prohibited.

The Possibilities of Rehabilitation

While society may have good reason to restrict the use of medical and behavioral interventions for "rehabilitation only" purposes, we can also believe that such interventions might be highly effective in changing the behavior of many offenders. To appreciate this possibility, it is important to recognize that the term "rehabilitation" can be defined in several ways. To some, it means helping offenders to stop committing crimes and to lead better lives. This is perhaps the most common definition of the term in the mind of the public. It implies some shift in the morality or psychology of offenders—in effect, a reformation. To others, rehabilitation may mean helping offenders to stop committing crimes, with the provision that whatever is done to them does not make their lives worse. Under this definition, some concern still focuses on the needs of individuals. To still others, rehabilitation might mean helping offenders to stop committing crimes without regard to whether their subsequent lives become any more or less gratifying. Under this definition, only society's goals are served and less concern extends to the individual. If the latter definition is adopted, then rehabilitation is not as elusive a goal as it might first seem. The psychological and physiological characteristics of offenders can simply be altered in ways that diminish their propensity to commit crimes. In reality, however, our societal values and legal and constitutional dictates govern what can be done—even when important social objectives are to be addressed.

If only societal needs are viewed as relevant, it would be possible to consider a number of ways of modifying the psychology and physiology of offenders to diminish their recidivism. Some are much more practical than others, but almost all that could be listed will, understandably, be troubling to most readers. They involve substantial invasions of the privacy of the minds and bodies of offenders. It has been suggested that the term "reconstruction" is more suitable than "rehabilitation" for these types of interventions (Ingraham and Smith 1972). All of the following interventions, however, further the societal objective of changing offenders in ways that diminish the risk that they will commit crimes and at the same time allow them to live in the community instead of in penal institutions.

1. *The "Clockwork Orange" scenario.* This proposal, based on a well-known novel and movie, involves the use of aversive conditioning to diminish violent or sexual behavior. The aversive stimulus must be an especially noxious chemical agent. Subjects can be exposed to their preferred antisocial activity and immediately receive a painful stimulus. (Something akin to this was tried at a state hospital in California when offenders were given the drug anectine after misbehaving.) Behaviorists doubt whether aversive conditioning alone can actually extinguish criminal behavior. It must be acknowledged, however, that aversive conditioning has never been implemented in a scientific way in a correctional or forensic institution. Ample evidence exists that, when utilized precisely and rationally, punishment can be a powerful modifier of behavior (Levis 1982). If instituted scientifically and with minimal regard for their well-being, it might be effective in modifying the antisocial behavior of offenders.

2. *Drug addiction.* If offenders could be deliberately addicted to a powerful narcotic drug, such as heroin, and the continued availability of that drug were made contingent upon law-abiding behavior in the free world, a certain number of offenders would probably settle for quiescent lives as addicts and abandon criminal behavior. As noted previously, this model could also be effective

in creating conformity in a controlled environment, such as a prison or hospital. Its influence in the "free world" might not be as powerful, but it would still contribute to the rehabilitation of many.

3. *Psychosurgery.* Serious and indiscriminate destruction of brain tissue would render almost any offender so incapacitated as to be unable to think or act with sufficient efficiency to engage in many forms of criminal behavior. Psychosurgery, however, can be more precise and less destructive. Sophisticated psychosurgical techniques have at times been used to ablate tiny areas of the brain believed to regulate violent behavior (Mark and Ervin 1970). Such surgery need not interfere with other social capacities of these offenders and could, at the same time, diminish their propensity for violent crimes. While the efficacy of these techniques has not been proven, good theoretical reasons exist for believing they would be effective (Elliott 1978).

4. *Antiandrogens.* Some evidence shows that the male sex hormone is associated with violence (Walker and Meyer 1981). Temporary chemical castration induced by antiandrogen drugs such as depo provera, in addition to alleviating the sex drive and thereby reducing sexual crimes, might also diminish the propensity of certain offenders to commit other types of violent acts.

5. *Neuroleptic medication.* Antipsychotic drugs, such as chlorpromazine, haloperidol, or fluphenazine, have powerful sedative and restraining effects on all individuals. Fluphenazine can be administered in depo form so that a single injection every 4 to 6 weeks will sustain its effects. Persons maintained on antipsychotic drugs have diminished tendencies for violence and would have considerable difficulty mustering the cognitive and motor skills required for criminal activity.

6. *"Brainwashing."* Placing subjects under conditions of great pain and deprivation, and then trying to change the nature of their ideology or belief systems, has had some effect in changing the orientation of prisoners in Communist nations. If the techniques are effective in making some persons abandon a capitalist ideology for a Communist belief system, they might also have some influence in increasing an offender's commitment to law-abiding behavior.

7. *Scientific operant conditioning programs.* If some offenders suffer from a defect that makes it more difficult for them than for normal people to develop conditioned responses, then a training program of precise and powerful operant conditioning, based on reinforcement as well as punishment, might help them learn to

conform (Eysenck 1977). (This may not be a true "rehabilitation only" approach, since it might remedy an actual defect.) Several programs of this type has been tried in the United States but have been abandoned because of lack of funds or because they have been vigorously protested by civil libertarians. A sound theoretical rationale supports this approach, however, and carefully designed programming might be quite successful (Burchard and Lane 1982).

Other scientific, but nonmedical or nonpsychological, technologies could be used to modify the behavior of offenders. These are even more alien to usual concepts of rehabilitation than those so far listed. Some offenders, for example, could be safely released from institutions if it were possible to keep close track of their whereabouts. It should be possible to use electronic "homing" devices to keep track of the whereabouts of offenders in community correctional programs through modern computer technology. Offenders who know they would be detected and apprehended once they left a certain area might be effectively restrained from committing certain types of crimes (Schwitzgebel 1969).

It can be argued that the listed interventions are not really aspects of rehabilitation but rather are better viewed as manifestations of chemical, surgical, or electronic restraint. Nevertheless, precedents apply for viewing most of them as rehabilitative techniques. Rehabilitation simply means restoration of individuals to a state of previous capacity. But it may also mean restoration to a state of health or freedom or to a capacity to work. Not infrequently, medical treatment that restores one capacity will restrain another. If patients who are psychotic are treated with antipsychotic medication, their capacities to make successful interpersonal accommodations may be restored, while other qualities, such as assertiveness or creativity, may be diminished. Individuals receiving antiandrogens can be restored to freedom and a crime-free life, although their sex life would be substantially diminished.

Some might insist that only spiritual or psychological reformation should be viewed as true rehabilitation. This is a very limited concept of rehabilitation, which assumes that change is a matter of volition or choice and excludes many medical interventions. It is preferable to view any intervention that restores an individual's capacity to live a noncriminal life in the free world as rehabilitative. Restraint is best considered an intervention, such as incarceration, that makes the commission of the physical aspects of most crimes impossible. (Admittedly, under these definitions, some interventions, such as amputating the hand of a pickpocket or electronic surveillance, would be difficult to classify.)

Overcoming Moral Objections to "Rehabilitation Only" Interventions

Some of the rehabilitative interventions I have discussed may seem rational and intriguing. Others may seem bizarre or barbaric. All would probably be rejected in our current social climate whether they were administered to offenders on a voluntary or an involuntary basis. "Rehabilitation only" interventions can be found ethically dubious on the basis of the following considerations:

1. Considerable doubt exists that any prisoner or inmate of a maximum security hospital can "volunteer" for a treatment when that intervention is held out as a means of gaining early release and the alternative to receiving it is continued incarceration. The issue here is whether prisoners or patients who live in a highly oppressive environment can ever give voluntary consent to treatments that may harm them.

2. A certain amount of crime, if not most crime, has political meaning. Where the motivation of criminal behavior is distinctly political, the use of interventions that change the thinking of offenders or compromise their physical capacities would significantly diminish the possibility of constructive as well as destructive dissent in society. Presumably, even political prisoners might become desperate enough while incarcerated to volunteer for treatments that would not only restore their access to society but destroy their capacity for dissent.

3. It is morally offensive to change the physiology and psychology of individuals as though they were objects or animals. In some instances, the interventions may be very painful. More often, they are degrading or compromise some aspect of the offender's humanity. Most of us view efforts to "tinker" with people's minds or to "alter" their brains as inherently inconsistent with the maintenance of a free society. Many would argue that the right of privacy and the right of free speech (and perhaps the right to generate ideas) granted by the first amendment offer even prisoners full protection from such degradations.

While these arguments are formidable, they are not insurmountable. We currently allow offenders to "volunteer" for certain interventions that have quite drastic biological consequences, such as receiving injections with antiandrogen drugs, which produce temporary castration. The argument that these interventions would diminish political dissent could be slightly muted by prohibiting offenders from volunteering for them until they receive detailed information about their consequences, including the possibility of loss of ideological commitment. It might be noted that we currently tolerate this risk without seeking informed consent when we impose psychotherapy on reluctant offenders for "rehabilitation only" purposes. The argument that these interventions are dehumanizing can be countered by weighing the morality of such dehumanization against the morality of imprisonment. It is legitimate to inquire whether forcing offenders to endure the pain, degradation, and suffering associated with spending 10, 20, or 30 years in prison is any less morally reprehensible than allowing offenders to submit to operations or to take drugs that would allow them to lead a life with certain limitations but in a free and relatively safe community. Civil libertarians might argue that prison is preferable, but it is unlikely that most offenders, if given full information about all options, would agree.

All of the hypothetical "rehabilitation only" interventions I have listed are "primitive," in the sense that they do not precisely control criminal behavior and they impose formidable restraints upon offenders unrelated to their capacities to engage in such behavior. It is unlikely that any of these interventions will be implemented in the near future. At some not too distant time, however, all of this is likely to change. As knowledge of the physiology and biochemistry of the brain increases, surgical, pharmacological, and behavioral techniques for changing behavior will become much more sophisticated. Using combined biological and behavioral therapies, it will be possible to diminish certain undesirable tendencies of offenders without drastically altering their human potentialities. At some point, when the harms imposed on offenders by "rehabilitation only" interventions are less than those created by incarceration, society may eagerly accept them. And, economic considerations will likewise be important: "rehabilitation only" interventions are far cheaper then incarceration.

The critical ethical issue of the future will be determining at what point the changes caused by "rehabilitation only" interventions are substantial enough and the harms negligible enough to justify their use. As the economic advantages of this response to crime become apparent to legislators, efforts may arise to create standards to permit their use, even when they remain ethically objectionable to many citizens. This is not a unique problem in our society. New scientific discoveries have forced us to face a host of complex issues related to the ethics of birth and death. Such issues as ovum transplants, genetic control, transplanting of body organs, and redefining the nature of death, all of which once seemed of interest only to those interested in science fiction, are now subjects of routine discussion in medicine. And, just as science has forced us to reconsider the ethics of birth, life, and death, it will inevitably force us to reconsider the ethics of crime, rehabilitation, and punishment. The ethical problems of rehabilitation will then be thrust upon us, whether we are ready to deal with them or not.

CHAPTER 9

Recommendations for Change

SOCIETY'S RESPONSE to the mentally disordered offender is but one aspect of society's response to the total issue of crime and punishment. Changes in any aspect of that response will have consequences for all aspects of the criminal justice system. Even minor changes in the manner in which we deal with mentally disordered offenders will have some impact on all other offenders. Conversely, changes in the manner in which the criminal justice system treats all offenders will directly influence the disposition of mentally disordered offenders.

In this chapter, I will consider two ways in which our system of criminal justice can be modified to provide more efficient and humane care to mentally disordered offenders. The first set of recommendations involves legal and policy changes that would directly influence how we deal with mentally disordered offenders. These recommendations, furthermore, would have only a minimal impact on other aspects of the criminal justice system. They are based on an assumption that the criminal justice system will continue to emphasize the desert/deterrence model and are entirely consistent with that model. The second set of recommendations is directed toward modifying the philosophical basis of our entire approach to criminal justice. I will argue that the criminal justice system should emphasize restraint/rehabilitation models over retributive models. The possibility of society's immediately initiating such changes is, of course, remote. Nevertheless, I am convinced that, with the passage of time, society will accept the restraint/rehabilitation model as the most humane, the most economic, and perhaps the most efficient approach to crime. To the extent that we move toward such a model, the specialness of the mentally disordered offender assumes less importance insofar as large numbers of offenders and perhaps the majority would be treated as though they were mentally disordered.

Changes in the Current System

Incompetent Offenders

Most of the policy and legal changes that would be helpful in our treatment of those found incompetent to stand trial have already been considered in other sections of this monograph. They will be briefly reviewed and discussed in the following:

1. *Evaluation of the offender's competency to stand trial should, wherever possible, be conducted in the community.* Only those offenders who have a history of violence or who appear to have a high probability of violence need to be evaluated in maximum security hospitals. Bail should be available for all other offenders whose competency is being evaluated. Many, if not most, evaluations could probably be done in an outpatient setting. Offenders who might require hospitalization for purposes of treatment only, and who do not need to be kept in a secure setting, should be treated in community hospitals.

This recommendation is slowly being implemented in many jurisdictions. Its more rapid implementation requires only a shift in policy or, in some states, minor changes in statutes to specify the locus of evaluation. Increased use of community evaluation would not diminish public safety. It would substantially expand the liberty of defendants evaluated for incompetency and make it easier for them to prepare their defenses.

2. *Evaluations of competency should be performed in as brief a period as possible.* In the community setting, only a few hours or days are necessary. In the maximum security hospital, 2 or 3 weeks should be sufficient.

Most jurisdictions are currently accelerating the process of evaluating competency to stand trial. It is difficult to know why we have, until recently, allowed this process to drag on for so many weeks or even months. Even when offenders spend many weeks in forensic hospitals, the amount of time they are actually evaluated by clinicians is often only a few hours. Conceivably something can be learned about the competency of offenders by observing their behavior on a day-to-day basis in the milieu of a security hospital, but what is learned is not likely to include the kind of information that is most critical for making the competency determination. It is possible that after offenders have spent weeks or months in such a milieu, their symptoms may be accentuated or diminished as a response to that particular environment. This change may tell the evaluator little about their capacities to proceed in the environment they will encounter when they return to trial.

To the extent that competency evaluations still are prolonged for periods of weeks or months, the criminal justice system should be viewed as responding to certain administrative needs of courts or institutions rather than to a need for accurate assessment. Briefer periods of evaluation would expedite the trial process and benefit both society and the offender. This goal could be realized with only minor administrative or statutory changes.

3. *Defendants who are sent to maximum security hospitals should, at the least, have copies of their arrest reports and indictments sent with them.* Previous medical and prison records should also be available to forensic hospital clinicians a day or two following admission. The delays many institutions now encounter in receiving these documents are inexcusable. They represent a form of bureaucratic inefficiency that compromises the quality of medical care and diminishes the accuracy of the evaluation process. If this simple requirement could not be mandated by administrative order, statutory change might be necessary.

4. *Clinicians who evaluate defendants for competency to proceed must be aware of their clients' rights.* Defendants should not be evaluated unless they already have attorneys who are aware of the circumstances of the evaluation. Defendants should be given a full explanation of the purposes of the clinical examination and of the potential uses of the report. Evaluators should carefully monitor their own use of therapeutic techniques, such as showing empathy, for the purpose of maximizing the defendant's self-disclosure. While the danger the defendant faces when examined by a mental health professional who is in a "double agent" role is now being scrutinized by our courts, this is an area where clinicians can also regulate themselves.

5. *For reasons discussed in chapter 3, mental health experts should not be allowed to testify in a conclusory manner that a defendant is either competent or incompetent to stand trial.*

6. *Attorneys should be made available to help clinicians determine a person's competency to proceed in the criminal process.* One of the criteria for competency to stand trial is the capacity to assist an attorney in one's own defense. Some clinicians know a great deal about legal proceedings and can judge what capacities

make a defendant more or less competent. Most, however, do not. It is probable that attorneys have many more skills in determining how well a client will assist them than clinicians. They also have a more precise idea of what demands they are likely to make on the offender in the course of a trial. If attorneys would spend at least one session together with mental health professionals, jointly interviewing defendants, the accuracy of the evaluation process would be significantly increased.

The major problem with this recommendation is the expense of implementing it. If the defendant has been sent to a geographically remote maximum security hospital, the defense attorney might not be available to assist the clinician. Neutral attorneys, less familiar with the case but certainly more objective, might have to be hired. It is likely, however, that whether neutral or defense attorneys were allowed to assist in the process of assessment, the ultimate result would be fewer judgments of incompetency. Returning more offenders to court would speed up the judicial process and might save society more than the cost of hiring additional attorneys. The increased accuracy of the evaluation process would benefit both society and the offender.

7. *Defendants found incompetent to stand trial should still have the opportunity to prove their innocence at a trial in which evidence unrelated to their competency can be presented (e.g., an alibi) or to challenge the adequacy of the indictment.* Greater efforts should also be made to try so called "unrestorable incompetents." The *Jackson* decision (*Jackson v. Indiana* 1972) protects most defendants from indefinite commitment, but it may allow for the release of some violent individuals who do not regain competency and who do not meet the criteria for civil commitment. Such cases involve a public safety issue, which can be resolved by bringing to trial offenders who have been committed as incompetent for a long period (6 months to a year) and who are not making progress toward recovery. At trial, they should be given the procedural safeguards recommended by Morris and others to help compensate for their incapacities (Morris 1982). However, since legal scholars continue to debate the constitutionality of bringing incompetent offenders to trial, this recommendation might be difficult to implement.

8. *Offenders who are found incompetent to stand trial should receive adequate psychiatric treatment and have access to learning experiences that will enhance their capacity to perform as defendants.* When defendants are not at high risk of committing violent

acts, their treatment should be conducted in the community, in either an outpatient or public hospital setting.

The Insanity Defense

Most of my opinions concerning the insanity defense have either been implied or expressed in chapter 4. Assuming that no change occurs in society's current retributive stance toward crime, it is difficult to envision how changes in the manner in which liability is assessed can have a major influence on protecting society or protecting the rights of offenders. Such changes might create more problems than they solve. Most of the following recommendations, therefore, are in the direction of sustaining the status quo and simply trying to make it somewhat more efficient and fair.

1. *The insanity defense should be retained.* By excusing a few, the insanity defense makes it easier for us to hold the majority of offenders responsible for their behavior. Such ascription of responsibility may also have utilitarian value, insofar as it facilitates efforts to change the behavior of offenders. If the insanity defense were abolished, the criminal justice system would also be likely to seek alternative means of mitigating the liability of the mentally ill. The impact of these new measures would be unpredictable. Various doctrines of partial responsibility (such as the diminished capacity doctrines) might be expanded and help create a situation in which sentencing and the ascription of responsibility would be even more inconsistent then they are now. With all of its reliance on anachronistic thinking, the insanity defense serves an important function in a society committed to retributive justice. If we wish to preserve the current system, we should learn to tolerate the expense and unwelcome outcome of some insanity cases and leave "bad enough alone."

2. *The standards used by various jurisdictions in determining insanity should be left intact.* There is currently a great deal of sentiment toward restricting the test of insanity to cognitive processes only and to delete the volitional test included in the American Law Institute standard. While volitional standards tend to be based on circular reasoning, it is hard to see what would be gained by eliminating them. They do allow juries a little more latitude in excusing persons who may be grossly impaired but whose cognitive functions are still intact enough to meet the *M'Naghten* stan-

dards for sanity. Furthermore, no evidence shows that including volitional standards has any real impact on the number of acquittals. The amount of legislative energy that would have to go into changing old or creating new standards would be considerable and would result in few, if any, benefits to society or to offenders.

3. *For reasons expressed in chapter 4, mental health experts should not testify in conclusory terms to issues of insanity.*

4. *For reasons expressed in chapter 4, the "guilty but mentally ill" verdict should be abolished.* It is simply a subterfuge that distracts the jury and society from dealing with the moral issue of criminal responsibility.

5. *Unless the insanity defense is viewed strictly as a mens rea defense (which requires proof of intent), the burden of proving insanity should be on the defendant.* It may be possible to prove intent beyond a reasonable doubt, but it is extremely difficult to prove sanity beyond a reasonable doubt.

6. *The testimony of mental health experts should be allowed in determining whether the offender's mental state at the time of a crime met the specific* mens rea *requirements for that crime.* Where the elements of a crime include mental states such as premeditation, deliberation, or malice, it is conceivable that some offenders (who would not be adjudicated insane) might be too mentally disturbed to have possessed them. Admittedly, however, this would occur rarely. (It should be clear that I am not recommending an expansion of the diminished capacity doctrine. Terms such as malice or premeditation should not be redefined to deal with the *capacity* to have a particular state of mind. I am merely arguing that existing law requires that all elements of the *mens rea* be proven beyond a reasonable doubt and that expert testimony may be relevant to the offender's actual state of mind.)

7. *Insanity acquittees should receive adequate psychiatric treatment.* Those who are unlikely to be violent should be treated in the community or in ordinary mental hospitals.

8. *Insanity acquittees who have been charged with violent crimes should be subject to careful social control.* Since the insanity defense is rarely invoked unless the crime has been committed, it can be assumed that those acquitted of violent crimes have engaged in violent behavior. Their release from forensic hospitals should be controlled by a parole board made up of behavioral and social scientists and community representatives. Mental health professionals should never be solely responsible for the release of insanity acquittees. When acquittees are released, they should be

subject to the same kind of parole monitoring required of other criminal offenders.

The foregoing recommendation is based on the public's concern that those acquitted of violent crimes by reason of insanity constitute a special danger to society. Given the knowledge that the best predictor of future violence is past violence, the public's anxiety is not entirely unfounded. The public has good reason to believe that insanity acquittees who have committed violent crimes have a higher probability of future violence than those ordinarily committed through civil procedures. If they are committed under the usual civil procedures, some will be prematurely released.

**Specialized Sentencing Programs
for Mentally Disordered Offenders**

The future of specialized indeterminate sentencing programs, currently embedded in a basically retributive system of criminal justice, is in doubt. With the lengthy sentences currently being given to so many sexual or "psychopathic" offenders, society hardly needs these programs for the protection they provide through restraint. The degree of protection society enjoys when and if some of these offenders are rehabilitated is also unclear. At the same time that the benefits of these programs to society are in doubt, it is apparent that they rarely provide adequate treatment for offenders and even impose formidable risks upon them. Indeterminately sentenced offenders may be incarcerated for longer periods of time than they would otherwise have been if sentenced under ordinary criminal codes. Even more disturbing, most of these programs are not truly indeterminate because they do not allow for early release as soon as rehabilitation is achieved. Accordingly, I would favor retention of these programs within our current system only if the following safeguards are offered:

1. *Offenders should not be committed to an indeterminate treatment program without the full benefits of procedural due process.* The standards that determine specialized commitment should also be precisely defined.

2. *A full range of treatment services should be provided for every offender indeterminately committed.*

3. *Release from an indeterminate program should be available at any time, even the day or week after admission.* To ensure this possibility, selected institutional staff should have the power to

recommend that an offender be considered for release at any time. A specialized review or parole board should have the power to enforce this recommendation.

4. *In the absence of institutional recommendations for release, offenders should still be entitled to a regular review for release consideration every 6 months.*

5. *Given the tendency of indeterminate programs to be characterized by ineffective treatment and conservatism regarding release, all offenders should have legal advocates.* Advocates should ascertain that their clients receive adequate treatment, that the case for their release is fully argued before parole boards, and that arbitrary refusals to release are challenged.

6. *Mental health professionals who help evaluate offenders for either determinate or indeterminate sentencing programs should conduct themselves in a manner that does not lead to unnecessary harm to offenders.* While the ethical guidelines for psychiatrists working in the legal process have already been noted, the following guideline is worth restating: *Experts should not testify in a conclusory manner as to whether a given individual is dangerous.* They should merely express their opinion as to the probability that a given antisocial act will occur in a given timespan and under certain conditions.

While only minor changes in policy or statute would be required to implement these recommendations, it is unlikely that items 2 to 6 would currently be acceptable in many jurisdictions. But if these changes are not accepted, I believe little would be lost by terminating current indeterminate programs. On the other hand, if these recommendations were to be implemented, I would favor expanding indeterminate sentencing, because it would bring us closer to the restraint/rehabilitation model advocated in the second part of this chapter.

Transfers

The issue of whether mentally disordered offenders are to be treated in prisons or in forensic hospitals is ultimately related to the conditions within those institutions. Harsh conditions within the prison increase the incidence of mental disorders among offenders. Harsh conditions and poor treatment facilities within forensic hospitals do not help mentally disordered offenders. Given the risks of stigmatization and loss of rights that offenders face when transferred, they are entitled to some quid pro quo in the form of treatment and decent living conditions. Within the current system, anything that would alleviate overcrowding and make prisons more humane and hospitals more therapeutic would significantly improve the plight of mentally disordered offenders who face transfer. It is particularly important that treatment standards in the prison and forensic hospital meet minimum requirements. Facilities for psychiatric treatment in prison should be no worse than those provided by community mental health centers in the average community. Treatment facilities in forensic hospitals should be no worse than those in public mental hospitals. These are not very high standards and do not call for the level of care currently available in the private sector.

Major Reform of the Criminal Justice System

While I have repeatedly questioned the fairness or practicality of the desert/deterrence model in criminal jurisprudence, it must be acknowledged that it is thriving in modern society. Much to the dismay of its more thoughtful advocates, it has also become a vehicle for society's vengeful motivations. When society is frightened by a perceived increase in crime, and when its citizens believe that severe punishment really does deter offenders, a desert/deterrence model is especially popular. Almost everyone these days, including many who consider themselves liberals, wants to "get tough" on crime. Most people now favor the death penalty, and executions are becoming more common. Compassion for offenders is at a low ebb. Even youthful offenders who were once sent to rehabilitation programs in relatively humane training school settings are increasingly tried as adults and given long prison sentences. Reform measures designed to cut down on the use of imprisonment are not seriously considered unless they are viewed as remedies for the overwhelming economic costs of imprisonment.

At the same time, the restraint/rehabilitation model enjoys little popularity. A significant amount of research has been interpreted as demonstrating that rehabilitation does not diminish offender recidivism. Offenders themselves have been described as wary of efforts to change their behavior and dissatisfied with indeterminate sentencing practices that leave them uncertain as to their release date. Libertarians feel that too many injustices involving highly intrusive treatments and prolonged sentences are inflicted upon offenders in the name of rehabilitation. Conservatives feel that rehabilitation leads to shorter time served in institutions and constitutes a lenient or "soft" approach to the criminal.

If any strong sentiment exists for rehabilitation these days, it is found among those who work in correctional settings. The idea that the keepers of prison inmates should simply restrain them and do nothing to try to change them is offensive to the dignity and sense of mission of correctional personnel. Wardens, educators, ministers, social workers, and psychologists continue to make sometimes heroic but usually unheralded attempts to rehabilitate their clients. Ironically, while the language of rehabilitation is rarely heard these days in the academic setting, it can still be heard quite regularly among those who spend their working days with prisoners.

The remainder of this chapter will present an analysis of the strengths and weaknesses of the desert/deterrence and the restraint/rehabilitation models, viewed in terms of the values of societal protection, justice or fairness, beneficence, and economy. Certain administrative approaches to crime, such as diversion (for reasons other than being mentally disordered) or restitution, will not be considered. These approaches, based on elements of both retribution and rehabilitation, do not currently have a major influence on the criminal justice system. (This is also a useful place to acknowledge that some might quarrel with my contention that the predominant model of criminal justice in the United States embodies the concepts of desert and deterrence. They might suggest that our current system could best be described as emphasizing desert and restraint. This viewpoint has some merit, but I believe that our society is highly committed to the deterrent value of punishment. At any rate, considerable historical and logical compatibility can be seen between the objectives of desert and deterrence and the objectives of restraint and rehabilitation.)

Which Model Provides Maximum Protection?

Great uncertainty is felt about the extent to which the desert/deterrence model protects society. It is reasonable to assume that it prevents a certain amount of crime related to private vengeance. At the same time, its general or specific deterrent value is questionable. The heavy emphasis on retribution in the past decade has been associated with only a minor reduction in crime rates. Even with much disagreement as to the validity of the FBI's Uniform Crime Reports as an index of the rate of crime, reported crime rates increased rather than decreased during the years of greatest emphasis on the justice model. (The very recent decrease in the crime rate is most parsimoniously explained by a corresponding decrease in the number of people in our society who are now reaching a crime-prone age.)

Scientific evidence has never supported the notion that invoking retribution more vigorously and more harshly would lower the incidence of crime. At best, the evidence that severity of punishment deters crime is inconclusive (Zimring and Hawkins 1973). It is more likely that the swiftness and certainty of punishment deters crime, but these goals are elusive in a society that advocates increasingly severe punishment (Nagin 1978). When the degree of punishment is harsh, offenders will only fight harder in the courts to delay it. Judges and juries will not convict unless evidence of guilt is substantial. To the extent that offenders fight more desperately to avoid punishment, its certainty becomes less likely.

Advocates of the desert/deterrence model have also argued that its use increases the likelihood that dangerous offenders will be kept safely in prison for longer periods than under a system of indeterminate sentencing. This argument assumes a high rate of inaccuracy in predicting the subsequent dangerousness of offenders released under an indeterminate model. It is usually buttressed by a "horror story" describing how a supposedly rehabilitated offender was released from an institution by a psychiatrist or parole board and subsequently committed an especially vicious crime. Violent crimes that are committed by individuals who could have been legally restrained may be exceptionally tragic and frustrating to society. They are certainly more noticeable than similar crimes committed by offenders who have been released after serving a fixed sentence. But the harm to society is likely to be similar, no matter what the circumstances of release. Under any model, almost all offenders who are not executed are ultimately released, and some of them will commit violent crimes.

No discipline concerned with criminology has developed criteria for determining when it is safe to release an offender. In the absence of any but arbitrary criteria, errors will be made and some dangerous people will be released. But the real issue here should be how frequently these errors occur, how much damage they impose upon the rest of society, and whether these errors are really any more destructive under one model of justice than another. A small amount of data compares subsequent crime rates for offenders released after a finding of not guilty by reason of insanity with crime rates of felons released after being convicted and imprisoned for the same crimes (Pasewark 1981). Although those found not guilty by reason of insanity are released much earlier, their crime rates tend to be identical to those of convicted felons. It is possible to conclude that the desert/deterrence response imposed upon convicted felons appears to provide no more protection than the restraint/rehabilitation response imposed upon insanity acquittees, even when the former response is directed toward "normal" offenders and the latter toward those adjudicated insane. Similar numbers of dangerous offenders appear to be released under any model of criminal justice.

In theory, the restraint/rehabilitation model should have an advantage in reducing dangerous crime by restraining all offenders until they are rehabilitated and can be safely released. The rehabilitative approach appears particularly attractive if we accept research findings indicating that a small number of offenders commit a disproportionate number of crimes (Wolfgang et al. 1972). It would seem that either rehabilitation or restraint of these persons would provide significant protection to the public. The most frustrating problem here is the lack of conclusive evidence that rehabilitation of these persons is possible with current technology (Martinson 1974). They may also be exceptionally persuasive in convincing therapists or parole boards that they have reformed, when in fact they are still at high risk of committing future violent crimes.

Other reasons make it doubtful that the restraint aspect of the restraint/rehabilitation model prevents as much crime as might be expected. A number of studies have indicated that reducing the length of imprisonment would lead to only a modest rise in the crime rate (Clarke 1974). An Ohio study has demonstrated that increasing restraint by sending all those indicted (not necessarily convicted) for a felony to prison for 5 years would reduce violent crime by only 4 percent (Van Dine et al. 1978). One reason for these unexpected findings is that new offenders, usually youth reaching the crime-prone age, simply assume the criminal careers of those who are restrained. Restraint is most likely to increase public protection when offenders who are at risk of being dangerous are identified while they are juveniles and kept imprisoned for long periods. Even if we knew how to identify which youth were at risk, it would be extremely difficult to find a constitutionally acceptable method of restraining them.

While the restraint/rehabilitation model may, in theory, provide more societal protection than the desert/deterrence model, no convincing evidence is available that it is currently able to do so.

Society must choose which of the two models to emphasize, knowing that neither model holds out much promise for protecting it and being unable to determine which is most efficient. Until predictive or rehabilitative techniques improve, we in effect have a "tie" between the two approaches. In this situation, society's choice should ultimately be determined by other values, such as fairness, beneficence, and economy. When both models are considered in terms of these values, it will be apparent that the restraint/rehabilitation model is the clear winner.

Fairness and Beneficence: The Desert/Deterrence Model

A major critique of the justice aspect of the desert/deterrence model I have alluded to throughout this monograph is that it is based on an indefensible view of human psychology. In assuming the sameness of most offenders, the model must of necessity reject much of the scientific data available regarding criminal behavior. Insofar as it treats people who have different degrees of blameworthiness, competency, and responsivity to punishment as though they were equal, it cannot be completely fair.

For the sake of argument, I will briefly repeat some material covered in other chapters relating to criminal liability and the differential responsivity of offenders to punishment. In dealing with an issue such as blameworthiness, the justice model assumes that people who do similar things in similar circumstances are equally punishable. This assumption can be maintained only by rigidly excluding most psychological evidence from the determination of the mental element (or *mens rea*) that defines a crime, and by ignoring biological and sociological differences that influence each individual's responsivity to social sanctions. The advocates of the justice model counter with the argument that, once we accept the deterministic arguments of science, we will end up accepting poorly documented theories, such as psychoanalysis, to explain everybody's behavior and thereby excuse everybody's behavior. But we do not have to resort to what is often unprovable psychoanalytic theory to point out the differences in people that influence their capacity or opportunity to adhere to law-abiding behavior. The new biological research and much of the old sociological research have shown substantial variability in the capacities for conditioning and opportunities for noncriminal behavior among those who regularly violate the law. Strong evidence is thus provided that people differ in their capacity to make the kind of benefit-risk evaluations involved in committing a crime with the degree of rationality the justice model assumes is present. If two individuals with differing capacities to avoid breaking a rule happen to break the same rule, it is not entirely fair to impose the same punishment upon them.

In dealing with punishment, the justice model also disregards the psychological effect of imprisonment on different individuals. In a truly just system, we would punish those who are equally liable, equally. Once imprisonment for a fixed period of time is used as the main form of punishment, this becomes impossible. People differ in their capacity to tolerate or survive imprisonment. A 10-week period of imprisonment may be a far greater punishment for one person than a 10-year period for another. If both are sentenced to 5 years of imprisonment for committing the same crime, they will not receive the same degree of punishment.

Factors other than the failure to deal with psychological variations should also lead us to question the fairness of current usages of the justice model. Even if we ignore the differential response of offenders to punishment and assume that all offenders are psychologically alike, the justice model is defensible as being fair only if it metes out the same punishment to all offenders who have committed the same crime under the same circumstances. In reality, such equality before the law is more an ideal than a fact in the United States. Offenders are treated unequally not as a response to their psychological differences (which might be fair), but as a response to their wealth.

Theoretical criminologists understand that crime must be defined not only in terms of the actors who commit illegal acts but also in terms of the processes by which certain acts are designated illegal (Quinney 1970). In short, crime cannot be understood solely by examining the behavior of the individual offender; the total context in which the society devises its prohibitions must also be examined. Unfortunately, the major schools of criminology that have focused on the societal role in defining crime have chosen to label their theories as Marxist or radical criminology. This has a negative impact on the appeal of their message, particularly at times when conservative attitudes are predominant. Radical criminologists also often confuse politics with data and use their observations to argue for social changes congruent with their personal views of a just society. But the data offered by the radicals (or by others who simply seek fairness) should nevertheless be sobering to anyone concerned with fairness.

To begin with, our society does not consistently define as criminal those acts causing the most harm to society. The criminal justice system focuses most of its attention on street crime and, to a lesser extent, on family crime. Relatively little attention is paid to corporate or white-collar crimes, which are generally committed by the more affluent. Corporate and white-collar crimes usually involve reckless conduct designed to create wealth and resulting in harm to others. The difference between this type of crime and street crime is the usual lack of intent to physically harm others, although taking the property of others may well be intended. If one leaves out the issue of intent, however, the amount of harm imposed upon our society by corporate or white-collar crime is probably greater than the amount imposed by street or family crime (Reiman 1979).

Definitions of crime that tend to protect middle and upper class groups are not the only factors that promote inequities in the criminal justice system. Considerable data regarding the incidence of crime in America suggest that the lower classes are especially likely to be punished. In various studies of arrest records of large populations of American boys, it has been noted that up to 50-60 percent are likely to be arrested for some nontraffic offense during their youthful years. Surveys in which persons are asked to report crimes they have committed, but which are never detected, reveal similar data about the ubiquitous nature of crime. It is likely that a majority of Americans have committed at least one crime (outside the field of legally prohibited sexual activities) without being detected. Many have committed crimes more than once. Much unreported crime is distributed uniformly throughout social classes and is far more serious than petty shoplifting. Workplace crime or theft by employees costs the American economy approximately $60 billion annually. Income tax fraud is also common, accounting for a loss of federal income in the United States estimated at over $60 billion annually (Reiman 1979).

With all of this crime, who gets punished? Only a small minority of offenders, say many. The late United States Senator Phillip Hart (1972) wrote:

Justice has two transmission belts, one for the rich and one for the poor. The low income transmission belt is easier to ride without falling off and it gets to prison in shorter order. The transmission belt for the affluent is a little slower and it passes innumerable stations where exits are temptingly convenient.

It should not be necessary to elaborate this point. Overwhelming evidence shows that, for the same criminal behavior, the poor are more likely to be arrested, more likely to be charged, more likely to be convicted, more likely to be sentenced to prison, and more likely to be given longer sentences than members of the middle and upper classes. Our current ruminations on the protocols of vengeance may not be relevant to the whole society. If all members of class A are sentenced fairly only with regard to other offenders in class A, but not with regard to offenders in class B or class C, the quest for fairness is fatally compromised. On this basis alone, the justice model as currently practiced may have a corroding effect on the moral sensibilities of the community.

It is fair to ask whether favoring the wealthy is an inherent aspect of the desert/deterrence model, or whether it would continue to occur even if we moved to a restraint/rehabilitation model. Undoubtedly, some individuals would continue to be advantaged and others disadvantaged under any system of justice. But one aspect of the desert/deterrence model tends to make these discrepancies worse. Because offenders will desperately seek to avoid the harsh punishment it inevitably imposes, the desert/deterrence model encourages an adversarial process at each stage of the criminal proceedings. Not only the determination of guilt but also the determination of the degree of punishment is likely to be contested. Thus far, our experience in using a restraint/rehabilitation model in dealing with the mentally ill suggests that it leads to a relatively small amount of litigation. In any contested legal proceeding, those who can afford to mount the best defense will be favored. To the extent society were to adopt a restraint/rehabilitation model, it is probable that fewer legal contests would ensue in which the wealthy would be more likely to prevail.

Intrinsic aspects of the desert/deterrence model also may diminish the likelihood that it will be used fairly or beneficently. Whenever this model has been in ascendancy, society's retributive impulses have been poorly controlled. Jeffery (1979) has suggested that punishing offenders is inherently reinforcing to the punisher. Viewed as aversive stimuli, offenders provide us with some sense of relief when we put them out of our way. If some offenders who are punished return to society and harm us again, we will soon become convinced that all offenders should be put away for longer periods of time. This kind of thinking ultimately results in prison overcrowding. As the quality of prison life diminishes, the probability increases that those who spend time in prison will come out more bitter and more antisocial than they were when they went in. When they commit new crimes, society's retributive impulses can again be justified and the process of excessive punishment continued in an almost self-perpetuating manner. This process is usually sustained until it is overridden, either by a sense of compassion for offenders or by its financial costs.

Unfortunately, the probability that the society that adheres to a desert/deterrence model will curb its retributive urges for beneficent reasons is remote. To the extent this model is not associated with rehabilitative efforts, it diminishes our capacity to feel compassion for offenders. If we do not try to change their behavior, we do not get to know them. Also, we tend not to identify or empathize with their suffering. Instead, we concern ourselves only with providing levels of care that seem humane and try to convince ourselves that we are treating them as they deserve to be treated. Those who are in daily contact with prisoners cannot, of course, fail to notice the suffering of offenders and to feel compassion for their plight. The efforts of correctional officials to try to change offenders' behavior, in addition to being motivated by needs to promote the stability of the institution, are also motivated by a benevolent wish to help them survive their current situation and learn to avoid future imprisonment. The beneficence of correctional workers, however, has only a tiny impact on the total force of society's commitment to retribution.

The process of escalating punishment in modern society is most likely to be slowed when its financial costs become unbearable. With so many offenders now imprisoned for such long terms, our society is very close to a point where it can no longer bear the financial burden of the justice/deterrence model. Two sources of expense are seen here. The first and most significant is the cost of imprisonment, which in some jurisdictions is up to $40,000 per offender per year. The second, a humanistic as well as a financial concern, is related to the waste of human resources associated with excessive use of prolonged imprisonment. Many currently imprisoned individuals would never commit a new crime if they were released. Some prisoners who would almost certainly be law-abiding and tax-paying citizens in the free world could be identified and released under a different model of justice.

Fairness and Beneficence: The Restraint/Rehabilitation Model

A restraint/rehabilitation model includes the possibility that some individuals who are not dangerous to society and who have committed only minor crimes may be imprisoned for very long periods. Their continued restraint does not protect society and forces them to endure undeserved suffering. When indeterminate

sentencing programs were more prevalent, "atrocity" stories describing the plight of prisoners locked up for decades were common. (These were the libertarian counterparts of "atrocity" stories
based on the premature release of dangerous offenders.) If we
were to return to a restraint/rehabilitation model, we would place
more offenders at risk of undeserved punishment. There is no way
to completely avoid this consequence as long as predictions of
dangerousness are so inaccurate with respect to both who should
be confined and who should be released. Given this risk of indeterminate sentencing, it must still be noted that the number of
offenders harmed by it is relatively small. As a rule, only minor
offenders are at special risk of spending more time incarcerated
under an indeterminate program than under a determinate sentence. On the whole, indeterminate programs have usually released
offenders earlier than determinate programs, and they have almost
always provided greater numbers of offenders with greater opportunities for freedom. This was true even in the days when civil
liberty attorneys were not available to protect offenders from arbitrary restraint. It should also be noted that indeterminate programs can reduce the likelihood that nondangerous offenders will
"rot" in prison by setting maximum sentences for certain nonviolent offenses and making only the minimum sentence indeterminate. Offenders convicted of violent crimes could continue to
receive indeterminate maximum sentences but have the right to
periodic review and legal advocacy for purposes of release.

The restraint/rehabilitation model has also been criticized as
unfair insofar as it leads to differing punishment for offenders
who commit the same crimes. Particularly when criteria for
determining when offenders should be released are unclear, patterns of release from indeterminate programs may appear discriminatory to many offenders. Those who are not released as soon
as others may understandably resent being retained in institutions
on the basis of their personal qualities rather than on the basis of
what they have done. This is an unfortunate and unavoidable consequence of the restraint/ rehabilitation model. It can be argued,
however, that discrimination on the basis of status is unlikely to
be avoided under any system of criminal justice. Under the justice
model, for example, inequities result when differences in psychological status are ignored in the process of imposing punishment.
Moreover, under any model, discrimination is possible on the basis
of wealth or influence. But discrimination based on evidence that

some offenders may be safely released sooner than others surely has sufficient utilitarian value to at least partially override moral objections to its existence. There would also appear to be some trade-off to offenders in the restraint/rehabilitation model that would diminish the more noxious aspect of this type of discrimination. That is, no matter how severe their crimes, all offenders have an opportunity for early release. And since all offenders can be provided equal access to treatment, this might in turn enhance the probability of their early release.

A related concern is that, under an indeterminate structure associated with the restraint/rehabilitation model, offenders suffer the uncertainty of never knowing when they will be released. Proponents of the justice model insist that inmates may be better off knowing they have a long sentence than facing the pains of indeterminacy, even when the latter form of sentencing is more likely to result in early release. This is one of those rare instances in which advocates of the desert/deterrence model seem to be concerned with the psychological suffering of offenders. But their concern with offenders' suffering in this instance is based on nothing more than "armchair" speculation. No one has systematically studied the extent to which offenders are actually damaged by having an unspecified release date. Nor has anyone even bothered to ask more than just a few offenders which system of sentencing they would prefer.

The rehabilitation model as applied to corrections has been criticized also because it allegedly puts inmates in a situation where they must prove to their keepers that they are ready for release. In the absence of any measurable criteria of change, according to this view, they may be forced to simulate improvement. Those who must decide when offenders are to be released then have the perplexing problem of evaluating whether the changes they observe are genuine or factitious. Usually they have no criteria to guide them. This can result in a kind of charade, in which offenders become preoccupied with using any device they can to prove to the staff that they have been rehabilitated, and the staff strives to avoid being fooled. Admittedly, this situation occurs frequently under the rehabilitative model. I would argue, however, that even at its worst this type of charade is unlikely to be harmful to either the inmate or the staff, and that it may even be helpful. The "games" involved in trying to prove that one is ready for release may be tedious and time consuming, but they hurt no one. Insofar as they provide hope, purposefulness, and a certain amount of excitement that distracts from the boredom of prison existence, the "games" may in fact be helpful to inmates. The very process of putting one's self into the patient or client role produces at least some behavioral change, and some of this change may be useful to the offender and to society. The correctional staff may, of course, be frustrated by the offender's manipulation, but this should not be a major issue. Persons who work with offenders must learn to deal with factitious behavior, and to the extent they understand it, their relationships with offenders and their skills as therapists will be enhanced.

The most serious objection to the restraint/rehabilitation model is the ethical one considered in the previous chapter. The model facilitates the use of biological and behavioral interventions for "rehabilitation only" purposes, with results that may help promote public safety but at the same time be distinctly disadvantageous to the offender and distasteful to our moral sensibilities. Rehabilitation, in short, may have malignant as well as beneficent consequences for offenders. It can be an oppressive weapon of a totalitarian state (as it sometimes appears to be in the Soviet Union), or it can be a caring and compassionate effort to help those who have put themselves in jeopardy of punishment. At present, the consciousness of our society with regard to rehabilitation is such that its use for repressive purposes would be discouraged. We also have an abundance of attorneys in our society who can be relied upon to protect the liberty interests of offenders. Thus far, these attorneys have successfully resisted efforts to use the most controversial forms of behavior modification or biological treatment to rehabilitate offenders. Meanwhile, those who might be unrestrained in inflicting behavior control upon offenders in pursuit of greater public safety still view rehabilitation as a way of "coddling" offenders and have not yet realized that certain "rehabilitation only" interventions would also serve social control purposes.

A danger always exists that the restraint/rehabilitation model will be used to further the interests of an oppressive state. However, as long as this tendency is controlled, and I believe it is controllable in the current political climate of the United States, the restraint/rehabilitation model is distinctly superior to the justice model in terms of fairness and beneficence. It is less discriminatory, imposes less pain on offenders as a group, and is especially merciful toward selected offenders who can be released when they are judged to be nondangerous to society.

A Word on Economy

We have every reason to believe that the restraint/rehabilitation model is superior to the desert/deterrence model from the standpoint of economy. First of all, it lessens the length of imprisonment and thereby cuts down on the rapidly escalating cost of imprisonment. Second, even if rehabilitation is only occasionally successful, those few successes save society the considerable expense of responding to the crimes rehabilitated offenders might otherwise have committed. Finally, the personnel and equipment costs required by current technologies of rehabilitation are relatively small when compared with the overall costs of providing institutional security. This situation will be somewhat altered as the technologies of rehabilitation become more sophisticated, but it is unlikely that the costs of implementing a rehabilitation program will ever exceed the cost of managing overcrowded prisons.

It should be pointed out, however, that one aspect of the desert/deterrence model that could, in theory, promote economy is capital punishment. If the legal costs involved in seeking and imposing the death penalty could be avoided, executing prisoners could certainly reduce the expenses of criminal justice. Utilitarian as well as moral reasons exist, however, for avoiding this solution. For one, it is unlikely that capital punishment deters crime. It is also probable that its existence creates an atmosphere in the correctional setting that is detrimental to the process of rehabilitation and increases the likelihood of prison violence. If the retributive actions of society are too painful, both prisoners and those who try to help them will find it difficult to sustain the qualities of mercy and hope associated with the process of social restoration. Prisoners become more angry and bitter. Many correctional officials I have known are against capital punishment, primarily because they believe its existence compromises their efforts to manage safe prisons.

Conclusion

Any criminal justice system is structured to serve retributive, deterrent, restraining, and rehabilitative purposes. I am not arguing that our criminal justice system should rush to abandon its commitment to desert and deterrence. I am simply advocating that we gradually put more emphasis on restraint and especially rehabilitation. This would mean more reliance on indeterminate sentencing, coupled with genuine efforts to provide adequate treatment for offenders and sincere efforts to protect their rights.

To the extent society moves toward a restraint/rehabilitation model, the classification and status of mentally disordered offenders would change. There would probably be some diminution in the use of the incompetency diversion. Attorneys and judges might be persuaded to lower the standard of competency or to seek competency evaluations less frequently if they knew convicted offenders would receive good treatment. It is also likely that the insanity plea would be raised less frequently, particularly if capital sentencing were not an issue and if acquittees were automatically institutionalized. When indeterminate institutionalization is the only alternative for the offender, whether acquitted by reason of insanity or convicted, the outcome of such acquittal would become much less attractive. To the extent all offenders were to be treated under an indeterminate model, programs for mentally disordered sex offenders or other allegedly dangerous offenders would be redundant. The need to transfer mentally disordered offenders to maximum security hospitals would also be significantly diminished if, under a rehabilitative model, prisons were able to offer adequate levels of treatment for all offenders.

I have tried to present both theoretical and practical justifications for the changes I have recommended. However, I have still one other reason for moving toward greater emphasis on restraint and rehabilitation as soon as possible. As the costs of criminal justice grow and the probability of finding relatively efficient, nonintrusive, and inexpensive means of changing behavior increases, a restraint/rehabilitation model is likely to be thrust upon us whether we welcome it or not. Society will then have to determine how repressive or humanistic the new criminal justice system will be. If we are to utilize new techniques coming out of the laboratory in a humanistic way, we must be fully aware of all the ethical and practical issues that will be raised by truly efficient rehabilitation based on biological and behavioral interventions. We should begin to seek such awareness while the ethical issues are still manageable.

REFERENCES

Abel, G.; Barlow, D.; Blanchard, E.; and Guild, D. The components of rapists' sexual arousal. *Archives of General Psychiatry* 34:895-903, 1977.

American Bar Association. *Criminal Justice Mental Health Standards*. Washington, D.C.: The Association, 1984.

American Law Institute. *Model Penal Code*. Philadelphia: The Institute, 1962.

American Law Institute. *Model Penal Code and Commentaries* (Official Draft and Revised Comments). Vol. 1. Philadelphia: The Institute, 1980.

American Psychiatric Association. *Clinical Aspects of the Violent Individual*. Task Force Report No. 8. Washington, D.C.: The Association, 1974.

American Psychiatric Association. *Diagnostic and Statistical Manual of Mental Disorders*, 3rd ed. (DSM-III). Washington, D.C.: The Association, 1980.

American Psychiatric Association. *Statement on the Insanity Defense*. Washington, D.C.: The Association, 1982.

American Psychiatric Association. *Issues in Forensic Psychiatry*. Washington, D.C.: The Association, 1984.

American Psychological Association. *Report of the task force on the role of psychology in the criminal justice system*. American Psychologist 33:1099-1113, 1978.

Andreasen, N.C., and Winokur, G. Secondary depression: Familial, clinical, and research perceptives. *American Journal of Psychiatry* 136:62-66, 1979.

Arenella, P. The diminished capacity and diminished responsibility defenses: Two children of a doomed marriage. *Columbia Law Review* 77:827-872, 1977.

Baker, S.L. Traumatic war disorders. In: Kaplan, H.; Freedman, A.; and Sadok, B., eds. *Comprehensive Textbook of Psychiatry*, Vol. III. Baltimore: Williams and Wilkins, 1980. pp. 1829-1841.

Baxstrom v. Herold, 383 U.S. 107 (1966).

Benson, H.; Beary, F.; and Carol, T. The relaxation response. *Psychiatry*. 37:37-46, 1974.

Bentham, J. *An Introduction to the Principles of Morals and Legislation* (1823 ed.). New York: Hafner, 1948.

Bloom, J.L., and Bloom, J.D. Disposition of insanity cases in Oregon. *Bulletin of the American Academy of Psychiatry and the Law* 9:93-99, 1981.

Bonnie, R.J. *A model statute on the insanity defense.* Charlottesville, Va.: University of Virginia Press, 1982.

Boslow, H.M., and Kohlmeyer, W.D. The Maryland defective delinquency law: An eight year follow-up. *American Journal of Psychiatry* 120:118-124, 1963.

Bowring v. Godwin, 551 F. 2nd 44,47,49 (4th Cir. 1977).

Brakel, S.J., and Rock, R.S. *The Mentally Disabled and the Law.* Chicago: University of Chicago Press, 1971.

Brodsky, S. Intervention models for mental health services in jails. In: Dunn, C.S., and Steadman, H.J., eds. *Mental Health Services in Local Jails*. National Institute of Mental Health. DHHS Pub. No. (ADM) 82-1181. Washington, D.C.: Supt. of Docs., U.S. Govt. Print. Off., 1982.

Brooks, A. *Law, Psychiatry and the Mental Health System.* Boston: Little, Brown, 1974.

Brown, B.S., and Courtless, T.F. The mentally retarded in penal and correctional institutions. *American Journal of Psychiatry* 124:1164-1166, 1968.

Burchard, J., and Lane, T. Crime and delinquency. In: Bellack, A.; Hersen, M.; and Kazdin, A., eds. *International Handbook of Behavior Modification and Therapy.* New York: Plenum, 1982.

Burt, R., and Morris, N. A proposal for the abolition of the incompetency plea. *University of Chicago Law Review* 40:66-95, 1972.

California Penal Code, 8 1026.1 (West Supp. 1981).

Chase, S. Where have all the patients gone? *Human Behavior* Oct. 1973, 2:14-21.

Churgin, M. The transfer of inmates to mental health facilities. In: Monahan, J., and Steadman, N., eds. *Mentally Disordered Offenders*. New York: Plenum, 1983.

Clarke, S. "Getting" em out of circulation: Does incarceration of juvenile offenders reduce crime? *Journal of Criminal Law and Criminology* 65:528-535, 1974.

Cleckley, H. *The Mask of Sanity.* 3rd ed. St. Louis: C.V. Mosby, 1955.

Clonce v. Richardson, 379 F. Supp. 338 (W.D. Md. 1974).

Cloninger, C.R.; Bonman, M.; and Siqvaldsson, J. Inheritance of alcohol abuse. *Archives of General Psychiatry* 38:861-868, 1981.

Collins, J.J., ed. *Drinking and Crime.* New York: Guilford Press, 1981. Comprehensive Crime Control Act of 1984 (Public Law 98-473).

Coury, J.J. Report of the Board of Trustees. American Medical Association Report G I-83, Chicago: American Medical Association 1984.

Delaware Code Ann. Title 11, 403(b) (1979).

Dix, G.E. Special dispositional alternatives for abnormal offenders. In: Monahan, J., and Steadman, H., eds. *Mentally Disordered Offenders.* New York: Plenum, 1983.

Donaldson v. O'Connor, 493 F. 2d 507 (5th cir., 1974).

Drope v. Missouri, 420 U.S. 162 (1975).

Durham v. United States, 214 F. 2d 862 (D.C. Cir., 1954).

Dusky v. United States, 363 U.S. 402 (1960).

Emmelkamp, H. Anxiety and fear. In: Bellack, A.; Hersen, M.; and Kazdin, A., eds. *International Handbook of Behavior Modification and Therapy.* New York: Plenum, 1982.

Elliott, F. Neurological factors in violent behavior (the dyscontrol syndrome). In: Sadoff, R., ed. *Violence and Responsibility.* New York: Spectrum, 1978.

Ennis, B. *Prisoners of Psychiatry.* New York: Harcourt, Brace, Jovanovich, 1972.

Ennis, B., and Embry, R. *The Rights of Mental Patients.* New York: Avon Books, 1978.

Ennis, B., and Hansen, C. *Memorandum of law: Competence to stand trial.* Journal of Psychiatry and Law Winter 1976, V: 491-514.

Estelle v. Gamble, 429 U.S. 97, 103 (1976).

Estelle v. Smith, 101 S. Ct. 1866 (1981).

Eysenck, H. *Crime and Personality.* London: Routledge and Kegan Paul, 1977.

Forer, L. *Criminals and Victims.* New York: Norton, 1980.

Frankel, M. *Criminal Sentences: Law Without Order.* New York: Hill and Wang, 1972.

Gardner v. Florida, 430 U.S. 349 (1977).

German, J.R., and Singer, A.C. Punishing the not guilty: Hospitalization of persons acquitted by reason of insanity. *Rutgers Law Review* 29:1076-1079, 1976.

Goldstein, A.S. *The Insanity Defense.* New Haven: Yale University Press, 1967.

Green, K. Psychological intervention. In: Green, K., and Schaefer, A., eds. *Forensic Psychology: A Primer for Legal and Mental Health Professionals.* Springfield, Ill.: Thomas, 1984.

Grostic, J.M. The constitutionality of Michigan's guilty but mentally ill verdict. *Journal of Law Reform* 12:188, 1978.

Groth, N. *Men Who Rape: The Psychology of the Offender.* New York: Plenum, 1979.

Groth, N. *Treatment of the Sexual Offender in a Correctional Institution.* Sommers, Conn.: Sex Offender Program, 1982.

Group for the Advancement of Psychiatry, Committee on Psychiatry and Law. *Misuse of Psychiatry in the Criminal Courts: Competency to Stand Trial.* New York: Group for the Advancement of Psychiatry, 1974.

Guttmacher, M., and Weihofen, H. *Psychiatry and the Law.* New York: Norton, 1952.

Guttmacher, M. A psychiatric approach to crime and corrections. *Law and Contemporary Problems* 23:633-649, 1958.

Guze, S. *Criminality and Psychiatric Disorders.* New York: Oxford University Press, 1976.

Guze, S.; Tuason, V.; Garfield, P.; Stewart, M.; and Picken, B. Psychiatric illness and crime: The role of alcoholism. *Diseases of the Nervous System* 29:239-243, 1968.

Halleck, S.L. *Psychiatry and the Dilemmas of Crime.* New York: Harper, 1967.

Halleck, S.L. *The Politics of Therapy.* New York: Science House, 1971.

Halleck, S.L. A troubled view of current trends in forensic psychiatry. *Journal of Psychiatry and Law* Summer 1974, II: 135-159.

Halleck, S.L. The assessment of responsibility in criminal law and psychiatric practice. In: *International Yearbook of Law and Psychiatry.* New York: Pergamon, 1984.

Halleck, S.L., and Witte, A.D. Is rehabilitation dead? *Crime and Delinquency* Oct. 1977, 23: 372-382.

Halpern, A.L. Use and misuse of psychiatry in competency examination of criminal defendants. *Psychiatric Annals* 5(4), 1975.

Hart, H.L. *Punishment and Responsibility: Essays in the Philosophy of Law.* New York: Oxford University Press, 1968.

Hart, P. Swindling and knavery, inc. *Playboy*, 19, Aug. 1972.

Hermann, D. *The Insanity Defense.* Springfield, Ill.: Thomas, 1983.

Hess, J.H. Incompetency proceedings, *Michigan Law Review* 59:1078-1100, 1961.

Illinois v. Lang, 76 Ill. 2d 311; 391 N.E. 2d 350 (1979).

Ingraham, B., and Smith, G. Electronic surveillance and control of behavior and its possible use in rehabilitation and parole. *Issues in Criminology* 7:35-52, 1972.

Jackson v. Indiana, 406 U.S. 715 (1972).

Jarvis, E. Criminal insane: Insane transgressors and insane convicts. *American Journal of Insanity* XIII:195-231, 1857.

Jeffery, C. *Criminal Responsibility and Mental Disease.* Springfield, Ill.: Thomas, 1967.

Jeffery, C. *Biology and Crime.* Beverly Hills: Sage, 1979.

Jones v. United States, 103 S. Ct. 3043 (1983).

Kadish, S., and Paulsen, M. *Criminal Law and Its Processes.* Boston: Little, Brown, 1975.

Kaimowitz v. Department of Mental Health. Unreported case. No. 73-19434-AW. (Cir. Ct. of Wayne County, Mich. July 10, 1973). Reprinted in Brooks, A.D. Law, Psychiatry and the Mental Health System. Boston: Little, Brown, 1974.

Kansas Stat. Ann. 22-3428b (1980 Supp.).

Kerr, C.A., and Roth, J.A. *A Study of Facilities and Programs for Mentally Disordered Offenders.* National Institute of Mental Health, in press.

Knecht v. Gillman, 488, F 2d, 1136 (8th Cir. 1973).

Kohlmeyer, W.A. The first year of operation under the new Patuxent Laws. *Bulletin of the American Academy of Psychiatry and the Law* 7:95-102, 1979.

LaFave, W.R., and Scott, A.W. *Handbook of Criminal Law.* St. Paul: West, 1972.

Lender, M.E., and Martin, J.K. *Drinking in America.* New York: Free Press, 1982.

Levis, D. Experimental and theoretical foundations of behavior modification. In: Bellack, A.; Hersen, M.; and Kazdin, A., eds. *International Handbook of Behavior Modification and Therapy.* New York: Plenum, 1982.

Lockett v. Ohio, 438 U.S. 586 (1978).

Mackey v. Procunier, 477 F. 2d 877 (9th Cir. 1973).

MacNamara, O. The medical model in correction, requiescat in pace. *Criminology* 14:439-448, 1977.

Mark, V.H., and Ervin, F.R. *Violence and the Brain.* New York: Harper & Row, 1970.

Marks, I.; Gelder, M.; and Bancroft, J. Sexual deviants two years after electric aversion. *British Journal of Psychiatry* 117:173-185, 1970.

Martinson, R. What works—questions and answers about prison reform. *The Public Interest* 35, Spring 1974.

Matthews v. Hardy, 420 F. 2d 607 (D.C. Cir. 1969).

McConaghy, N. Sexual deviation. In: Bellack, A.; Hersen, M.; and Kazdin, A., eds. *International Handbook of Behavior Modification and Therapy.* New York: Plenum, 1982.

McDonald, J. *The Murderer and His Victim.* Springfield, Ill.: Thomas, 1961.

McGarry, A.L.; Curran, W.J.; Lipsett, P.D.; Lelos, D.; Schwitzgebel, R.K.; and Rosenberg, A.H. *Competency to Stand Trial and Mental Illness.* Final Report. National Institute of Mental Health. DHEW Pub. No. (HSM) 73-9105. Washington, D.C.: Supt. of Docs., U.S. Govt. Print. Off., 1973.

McGarry, L., and Bendt, R. Criminal v. civil commitment of psychotic offenders: A seven year follow-up. *American Journal of Psychiatry* 125:193-201, 1969.

Mednick, S., and Hutchings, B. Some considerations in the interpretation of the Danish adoption studies. In: Mednick, S., and Christiansen, K., eds. *Biosocial Basis of Criminal Behavior.* New York: Gardner Press, 1977.

Mednick, S., and Volavka, J. Biology and crime. In: Morris, N., and Tonry, M., eds. *Crime and Justice, An Annual Review of Research.* Chicago: University of Chicago Press, 1980.

Meehl, P. *Psychodiagnosis: Selected Papers.* Minneapolis: University of Minnesota Press, 1973.

Megargee, E. The prediction of dangerous behavior. *Criminal Justice and Behavior* 3:3-21, 1976.

Menninger, K. *Verdict guilty—now what?* Harper's Magazine 199, Aug. 1959.

Menninger, K. *The Crime of Punishment.* New York: Viking Press, 1968.

M'Naghten's Case, 10 Clark and Fin. 200, 8 Eng., Rep. 718 (1843).

Monahan, J. *The Clinical Prediction of Violent Behavior*. National Institute of Mental Health. DHHS Pub. No. (ADM)81921. Washington, D.C.: Supt. of Docs., U.S. Govt. Print. Off., 1981.

Monahan, J., and Davis, S. Mentally disordered sex offenders. In: Monahan, J., and Steadman, H., eds. *Mentally Disordered Offenders*. New York: Plenum, 1983.

Monahan, J.; Caldeira, L.; and Priedlander, A. Police and the mentally ill: A comparison of committed and arrested persons. *International Journal of Law and Psychiatry* 2:509-518, 1979.

Monahan, J.; Davis, S.; Hartstone, E.; and Steadman, H. Prisoners transferred to mental hospitals. In: Monahan, J., and Steadman, H., eds. *Mentally Disordered Offenders*. New York: Plenum, 1983.

Monahan, J., and Steadman, H. Crime and mental disorders: An epidemiological approach. In: Morris, N., and Tonry, M., eds. *Review of Research in Crime and Justice*. Chicago: University of Chicago Press, 1982.

Monahan, J., and Steadman, H. *Mentally Disordered Offenders*. New York: Plenum, 1983.

Morris, G. Acquittal by reason of insanity. In: Monahan, J., and Steadman, H., eds. *Mentally Disordered Offenders*. New York: Plenum, 1983.

Morris, N. *The Future of Imprisonment*. Chicago: University of Chicago Press, 1974.

Morris, N. *Madness and the Criminal Law*. Chicago: University of Chicago Press, 1982.

Mowbray, C. A study of patients treated as incompetent to stand trial. *Social Psychiatry* 14:31-39, 1979.

Nagin, D. General deterrence: A review of the empirical evidence. In: Blumstein, A.; Cohen, J.; and Nagin, D., eds. *Deterrence and Incapacitation: Estimating the Effects of Criminal Sanctions on Crime Rates*. Washington, D.C.: National Academy of Sciences, 1978.

O'Connor v. Donaldson, 422 U.S. 563 (1975).

Parker, M. California's new scheme for the commitment of individuals found incompetent to stand trial. *Pacific Law Journal* 6:484, 1975.

Pasewark, R. The insanity plea: A review of the research literature. *Journal of Psychiatry and Law* 9:357-401, 1981.

Pate v. Robinson, 383 U.S. 375 (1966).

Pearson v. Probate Court, 309 U.S. 370 (1940).

People v. McQuillan, 392 Mich. 511, 221 N.W. 2d 569 (1974).

Perkins, D. Assessment and treatment of dangerous sexual offenders. In: Hinton, J., ed. *Dangerousness: Problems of Assessment and Prediction.* London: Allen and Unwin, 1983.

Perkins, R. *Perkins on Criminal Law.* 2d ed. Mineola, N.Y.: The Foundation Press, 1969.

Quinney, R. *The Social Reality of Crime.* Boston: Little, Brown, 1970.

Rabkin, J. Criminal behavior of discharged mental patients: A critical appraisal of the research. *Psychological Bulletin* 86:1-27, 1979.

Radin, M.J. Cruel punishment and respect for persons: Super due process for death. *Southern California Law Review* 53:1143-1185, 1980.

Rawls, J. *A Theory of Justice.* Cambridge: Harvard University Press, 1971.

Reiman, J.H. *The Rich Get Richer and the Poor Get Prison.* New York: Wiley, 1979.

Rennie, Y. *The Search for Criminal Man.* Lexington, Mass.: Heath, 1978.

Rennie v. Klein, 462 F. Supp. 1131 (D.N.J., 1978)

Robey, A. Criteria for competency to stand trial: A checklist for psychiatrists. *American Journal of Psychiatry* 122:612622, 1965.

Robitscher, J. *The Powers of Psychiatry.* New York: Houghton Mifflin, 1980.

Roesch, R., and Golding, S.L. *A systems analysis of competency to stand trial procedures: Implications for forensic services in North Carolina.* Urbana, Ill.: University of Illinois Press, 1977.

Roesch, R., and Golding, S.L. *Competency to Stand Trial.* Urbana, Ill.: University of Illinois Press, 1980.

Rogers, J.L. Oregon legislation relating to the insanity defense and the Psychiatry Security Review Board. *Willamete Law Review* 18:23-48, 1982.

Rogers v. Okin, 634 F. 2d (1st Cir. 1980).

Roth, L.H. Correctional psychiatry. In: Curran, W.S.; McGarry, A.L.; and Perry, C.S., eds. *Modern Legal Medicine, Psychiatry and Forensic Science.* Philadelphia: Davis, 1980.

Rouse v. Cameron, 373 F. 2d. 45 (D.C. Cir. 1966).

Sarbin, T. The dangerous individual: An outcome of social identity transformations. *British Journal of Criminology* 7:285-293, 1967.

Schuster v. Herold, 410 F. 2d 1071, 1090 (2d. Cir. 1969).

Schwartz, S.A. Moving backward confidently: Michigan's new laws on criminal responsibility. *Michigan State Bar Journal* 54:817-904, 1975.

Schwitzgebel, R. A belt from big brother. *Psychology Today* 2(11):45-47, 1969.

Scull, A. *Decarceration, Community Treatment and the Deviant: A Radical View.* Englewood Cliffs, N.J.: Prentice-Hall, 1977.

Shah, S.A. Some interactions of law and mental health in the handling of social deviance. *Catholic University Law Review* 23:674-719, 1974.

Shah, S.A. Criminal responsibility. In: Curran, W.J.; McGarry, A.L.; and Shah, S.A., eds. *Forensic Psychiatry and Psychology.* Philadelphia: F.A. Davis, 1986.

Shah, S.A. Dangerousness: A paradigm for exploring some issues in law and psychology. *American Psychologist* 33:224-238, 1978.

Shupe, L. Alcohol and crime. *Journal of Criminal Law and Criminology* 44:661-664, 1954.

Sieling v. Eyman, 478 F. 2d 211 (9th Cir. 1973).

Siever, L.J. Biogenetic factors in personalities. In: Frosch, J.P., ed. *Current Perspectives on Personality Disorders.* Washington, D.C.: American Psychiatric Press, 1983.

Silberman, C.E. *Criminal Violence, Criminal Justice.* New York: Random House, 1978.

Singer, P. Sending men to prison: Constitutional aspects of the burden of proof and the doctrine of the least drastic alternative as applied to sentencing determinations. *Cornell Law Review* 58:51-72, 1972.

Slovenko, R. *Psychiatry and Law.* Boston: Little, Brown, 1973.

Slovenko, R., and Luby, E. From moral treatment to railroading out of the mental hospital. *Bulletin of the American Academy of Psychiatry and the Law* 4:223-236, 1974.

Specht v. Patterson, 386 U.S. 605 (1967).

Spieker, G., and Sarver, R. Alcohol and crime. *British Journal on Alcohol and Alcoholism* 134:184-189, 1979.

State v. Hayes, 389 A. 2d 1379 (N.H. 1978).

State v. Krol, 68 N.J. 236, 344 A 2d 289 (1975).

State v. Little, 199 Neb. 772, 261 N.W. 2d 847 (1978).

Steadman, H. *Beating a Rap.* Chicago: University of Chicago Press, 1979.

Steadman, H. Critically reassessing the accuracy of public predictions of the dangerousness of the mentally ill. *Journal of Health and Social Behavior* 22:310-316, 1981.

Steadman, H.J., and Braff, S. Defendants not guilty by reason of insanity. In: Monahan, J., and Steadman, H.J., eds. *Mentally Disordered Offenders*. New York: Plenum, 1983.

Steadman, H.J., and Hartstone, E. Defendants incompetent to stand trial. In: Monahan, J., and Steadman, H.J., eds. *Mentally Disordered Offenders*. New York: Plenum, 1983.

Steadman, H.J.; Vanderwyst, D.; and Ribner, S. Comparing arrest rates of mental patients and criminal offenders. *American Journal of Psychiatry* 135:1218-1220, 1978.

Stone, A. *Mental Health and Law: A System in Transition*. National Institute of Mental Health. DHEW Pub. No. (ADM)75176. Washington, D.C.: Supt. of Docs., U.S. Govt. Print. Off., 1975.

Stone, A. The right to treatment and the psychiatric establishment. In: Bonnie, R., ed. *Diagnosis and Debate*. New York: Insight Communication, 1977.

Strong, S.L. Social psychological approach to psychotherapy research. In: Garfield, S.L., and Bergin, A.E., eds. *Handbook of Psychotherapy and Behavior Change*. 2d ed. New York: Wiley, 1978.

Sturup, G. Castration: The total treatment. In: Resnick, H., and Wolfgang, M.E., eds. *Sexual Behavior*. Boston: Little, Brown, 1972.

Sutherland, E.H. The diffusion of sexual psychopath laws. *American Journal of Sociology* 56:142-148, 1950.

Sykes, G. *The Society of Captives*. Princeton, N.J.: Princeton University Press, 1958.

Szasz, T. *Law, Liberty and Psychiatry*. New York: Macmillan, 1963.

Szasz, T. *Ideology and Insanity*. Garden City, N.Y.: Doubleday, 1972.

In re Thompson, 362 N.E. 2d 532 (Mass. App. 1977).

Thurrell, R.; Halleck, S.; and Johnson, A. Psychosis in prison. *Journal of Criminal Law, Criminology, and Police Science* 4:271, 276, 1965.

Toch, H. *Living in Prison*. New York: Free Press, 1977.

Toch, H. Psychological treatment of imprisoned offenders. In: Hays, S.; Roberts, T.; and Solway, K., eds. *Violence and the Violent Individual*. New York: SP Medical and Scientific Books, 1981.

Vaillant, G.E., and Perry, J.C. Personality disorders. In: Kaplan, H.; Freedman, A.; and Sadok, B., eds. *Comprehensive Textbook of Psychiatry III*. Vol. 2. Baltimore: Williams and Wilkins, 1980.

Van Dine, S.; Dinitz, S.; and Conrad, J. The incapacitation of the dangerous offender: A statistical experiment. In: Conrad, J., and Dinitz, S., eds. *In Fear of Each Other*. Lexington, Mass.: Lexington Books, 1978.

Vitek v. Jones, 445 U.S. 480, 100 S.Ct. 1254 (1980).

Walker, N., and McCabe, S. *Crime and Insanity in England*. Scotland: Edinburgh University Press, 1973.

Walker, P., and Meyer, W. Medroxyprogesterone acetate treatment for paraphiliac sex offenders. In: Hays, J.; Roberts, T.; and Solway, K., eds. *Violence and the Violent Individual*. New York: SP Medical and Scientific Books, 1981.

Wexler, D. *Criminal Commitments and Dangerous Mental Patients: Legal Issues of Confinement and Release. National Institute of Mental Health*. DHEW Pub. No. (ADM)76-28650. Washington, D.C.: Supt. of Docs., U.S. Govt. Print. Off., 1976.

Wexler, D. Token and taboo: Behavior modification, token economics, and the law. *California Law Review* 61:81-109, 1973.

Whitaker, C. *The Family Crucible*. New York: Harper and Row, 1978.

Wieter v. Settle, 193 F. Supp. 318 (W.D. Mo. 1968).

Winick, B.J. Psychotropic medication and competence to stand trial. *American Bar Foundation Research Journal* 76:9-816, 1977.

Winick, B.J. Incompetence to stand trial: Developments in the law. In: Monahan, J., and Steadman, H.J., eds. *Mentally Disordered Offenders*. New York: Plenum, 1983.

Winick, B.J., and Demo, T.L. Competence to stand trial in Florida. *University of Miami Law Review* 35:31-76, 1980.

Wojtowicz v. United States, 550 F. 2d 786 (2d Cir. 1977).

Wolfgang, M.E.; Figlio, R.M.; and Sellin, T. *Delinquency in a Birth Cohort*. Chicago: University of Chicago Press, 1972.

Woodruff, R.; Goodwin, D.; and Guze, S. *Psychiatric Diagnosis*. New York: Oxford University Press, 1974.

Wootton, B. Book Review of Goldstein, A., *The Insanity Defense*. *Yale Law Journal* 77:102.7–1032, 1968.

Zimring, F., and Hawkins, G. *Deterrence*. Chicago: University of Chicago Press, 1973.